BE THE JAGUAR YOU ALWAYS WANTED TO BE

KEEP MOVING AND LIVE YOUR BEST LIFE

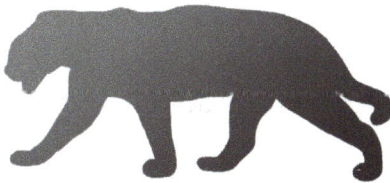

DR. EMMANOUIL (MANOS) GEORGIADIS

EU Conformity Declaration

This product complies with the following safety regulations and standards to ensure consumer safety and product quality: Regulation (EU) 2023/988 of the European Parliament and of the Council on General Product Safety (GPSR): The Consumer Product Safety Improvement Act (CPSIA), Section 101. The Californian Safe drinking water and toxic enforcement act. (Proposition 65) EN71-Part 1: Mechanical and Physical Properties EN71-Part 2: Flammability EN71-Part 3 Migration of certain elements.

Published and Manufactured by Softwood Books
EU Responsible person: Maddy Glenn
Office 2, Wharfside House, Prentice Road, Stowmarket, Suffolk, IP14 1RD
www.softwoodbooks.com
hello@softwoodbooks.com

EU Rep:
Authorised Rep Compliance Ltd., Ground Floor, 71 Lower Baggot Street, Dublin, D02 P593, Ireland
www.arccompliance.com
info@arccompliance.com

Paperback ISBN: 978-1-0369-0614-6

To my parents and brothers. Without your constant support and care, nothing would have been possible.

Contents

FOREWORD 1   6

FOREWORD 2   7

INTRODUCTION   9

We and Our Loved Ones   18

The Evolution   20

The Substances   23

The Stroll   30

The Magic Lake   35

Dopamine   40

Avoiding the Magic Lake   42

How Much Exercise Do You Need?   46

Reduced Physical Activity   53

The New Habit   55

The Benefits of Frequent Physical Activity   61

Epigenetics and Physical Activity   80

Why You're Avoiding Physical Activity   83

What Prevents and What Enhances Regular Physical Activity?   86

10 + 1 Questions and Answers   103

A Few Words at the End   114

Bibliography   115

About the Author — Acknowledgements   125

FOREWORD 1

I am really happy to write this foreword for lots of reasons. The main reason is the author himself. He's one of those people who serve their science by example. Apart from being friends, Manos Georgiadis and I have worked together professionally at the Greek Police Officers' School, and I've found that his thinking and actions are oriented towards improving quality of life. In this book, he brings together the clarity of scientific writing and the detail of documentation, with the immediacy and vividness of narrative. He expresses what he has been advocating for years, through his own experience; the benefits of a motivated body.

He writes about all kinds of interesting things, like the internet, how we can change our habits, and the challenges of artificial intelligence. He also talks about the effects of the environmental crisis on our bodies and minds. He even uses examples from the recent pandemic to show how we can take better care of ourselves. It's clear to me that the experience of the pandemic has shown us all that we need to take a good, hard look at the modern way of life. This book is full of useful advice, like how much and what kind of physical activity each age group needs, as well as advice for people living with chronic diseases and disabilities. We'll dive into the motivation for physical activity, and the benefits of its frequency, through some questions we're all concerned with in relation to physical activity. So, reading this book, I was reminded of Manos's wonderful verbal advice on all these things. Having walked the path of exercise and sport psychology himself for many years now, I believe that with this book he expresses his mature desire to share the knowledge he has gained, in a comprehensible and motivating way, to all human beings. And he is greatly successful!

Nikos Houtas, Ph.D. in Modern History

FOREWORD 2

When born we may not know whether we'll inherit any property from our parents, but we do know that we'll inherit neuroses and diseases.

We all have a unique set of experiences that we've accumulated over the years. Some of us are born into more fortunate circumstances, while others may face challenges along the way. These experiences are passed down through our genes and shape our lives in ways we may not even realize. Our past is extended by our grandparents and, of course, our parents. It's so sad when negative attitudes and psychological traumas are passed on to offspring, creating behaviors that are often hard to justify. So, the environment around us will then take over this role. It'll decide whether our genes are expressed or not, and how they're affected by things like family, the people we meet, and even the part of the planet we're born into.

It's clear that our behaviors affect our physical, mental, and spiritual health. And so, we find ourselves in situations that aren't so pleasant, and we feel like we can't change them. But is that true?

Have you ever wondered if our lives could change drastically at certain sedentary periods of time, due to an illness or an accident? Many would describe these as negative periods in life. Periods that luck played a big part in the conditions we find ourselves in.

Apart from the instants when events happen to us, there are also difficult moments when we are called upon to decide. It's often in the toughest times that we must make the most important decisions.

And it's the decisions we make in those tough and pivotal moments that really matter. They can either lead us to the next rough patch, or help us grow and evolve in ways that benefit us in the long run.

No matter how daunting things get, it's a chance to stand up and decide how to move forward. You can't change the past, but you can sure as heck destroy the present by not acting on it! Get stuck on everything that has happened in your life so far, and you'll never move forward. It doesn't matter how many times you fall, if you get up one more time. And if you do that, then you've certainly achieved more than you had before.

Self-care is something we all need, but it's not usually something we're taught when we're young. However, it relates to knowledge we can learn as we go along — and it can help in every area of our lives.

So, this is your moment! With the book you hold in your hands, you'll find the ability to determine your future and make important decisions for your life to improve.

Dr Emmanouil (Manos) Georgiadis is an amazing individual with an incredible enterprising spirit. In this book, he'll show you how to chart your own path and succeed in every area of your life. You'll discover how small changes in your daily routine can lead to big results. All you need to do is invest your time wisely, and establish little nuggets of discipline with these wonderful things you'll learn. And don't forget:

It's widely known that personal discipline isn't always easy to embrace. But, as they say, the proof of the pudding is in the eating. The results speak for themselves.

Evangelos Zoubaneas

Nutritionist, Author, Director of Education & Training Centre Response

Eating Disorders (www.keadd.gr)

INTRODUCTION

It's so easy to find important information about any hobby, activity, scientific field, or personal needs just by pressing Enter on the search box of your PC or, even easier, your smartphone. However, it can be tricky to find reliable information online. It takes time to know where to look and what to search for.

So, as there's so much available information and your time is limited, where do you start? How do you decide where to search? How do you pick the most reliable sources based on your interests? And how do you narrow down the information you find (this last one is perhaps the most important, due to the plethora of information available on the internet)? In other words, how do you find the most interesting or useful information each time you want to take an informed decision?

When things get little tricky, social networks often come to the rescue. They seem to have just the right amount of information, without overwhelming us with other "useless" information that — due to complexity or lack of expertise — we can't handle. Thanks to our registered interests and based on friends and like-minded people, we can learn about the subjects which interests us, in quick and simple ways, and in a language we understand. We can also add our own thoughts and feelings if we want to, which makes the whole process even more fun.

Isn't it great how social networks make everything easy and simple? A wise algorithm takes care of this by excluding content that I dislike or find uninteresting, which is great because it means I can focus on the things I want to read or watch. I don't have to spend my precious time reading long texts or watching long lectures. I can just read the opinions and possible debates that interest me. Most of the time, the message is simple; it might be about a wonderful new product that promises miracles but it's always easier to access the information, so I can get a basic view on what I'm concerned about. The new Artificial

Intelligence (AI) machines are also brilliant in enhancing this experience by offering abstracted information on the subject I am looking at. Isn't it great?

Maybe not.

Okay, I'm not an expert, but I feel like I've got the basics down. I'm not going to be taking an exam on the subject, so I'm not too worried about it. I may not be the smartest person in the world, but I do know that most people agree on the basics. And of course, we all think logically. I'm so happy to say that my friends and acquaintances agree with me on this! It's as simple as that.

I think the main problem with these searches is that any obtained information does not really register. Or it isn't really understood, apart from its basics. It's so easy to digest, but it doesn't really stick in my mind. As easy it is to access it, with the same speed any new data quickly vanishes from my brain. Hence, this knowledge can't be used to change my behavior according to my personal goals and decisions.

On the other hand, like everyone else, I get really excited about stories and narratives that have a beginning, middle, and end. A plot that makes sense and a progression that I can follow (Yuval Noah Harari, (2015). Sapiens: A Brief History of Humankind). Through them, I've been able to communicate, collaborate, evolve, and even survive on this unpredictable and difficult-to-inhabit planet.

Stories helped me learn how to work with others and achieve my goals. Stories help me understand myself and the world around me. Stories are important to me because they help me make sense of the world and keep me engaged. I love how they have plots, twists, and turns that give meaning and continuity.

This book is here to answer many of your questions. It offers a story that helps you think about the basics of life and how you can make it better. And it gets you thinking about the most essential human behavior: how you live connected with your physical self, the ways you move your body, and how you take care of yourself.

Without having any limits, worries, or stressors. Just for you and your experience. Every single day, without any comparisons or circumstances that might get in the way of enjoying this practice.

When one thinks about the challenges in today's society, it's important to remember how crucial physical activity is for a happy and healthy life.

The first and most important thing one can do today is to try to maintain a good mental state and a positive mood. It's essential to find a way to balance all the demands of daily living, using options that create a feel-good effect, providing a chance to relax and improve mental health.

It can be tricky to keep a good balance between what one wants and whatever one's obligations are, and — apparently — the faster one goes, the harder this balance is. However, I'm happy to suggest that the more one connects to one's own body functions, the more achievable it is to balance psychological, physical, and cognitive needs, making decisions that enhance one's health.

Another challenge in today's society is technology and how it affects one's daily life. Every new technological development offers new solutions and possibilities aimed at improving life — which is great — but at the same time, it makes daily life a little more intricate, with all the different complications that creates.

Take computer games, for instance. They offer so many new possibilities for entertainment and learning, and many of their applications have provided new solutions to medicine, engineering, and education. At the same time, however, they can have a negative effect on children's social skills, as well as their motor and physical development. It's so sad to see how much time kids and adolescents are spending in front of screens nowadays. Traditional play activities like running around, playing 'it', and climbing trees are becoming a thing of the past. This doesn't help the developing child's brain at all. It has lots of negative effects on things like strength, speed, balance, and endurance. It also affects how well children can perceive things in three dimensions.

It's quite simple: a child's brain — until the age of nine or ten years — just can't develop and evolve without daily, long-lasting playtime that involves a variety of physical activities like bouncing, kicking, climbing, running, and balancing.

I wonder how many parents are aware of this; I'd love to know!

Now, let me switch gears and talk about the internet. It's changed my habits in so many ways. It's so great that the internet and its related apps have enabled billions of people to keep working during the recent pandemic. At the same time, though, it has changed professional circumstances forever. It was a real eye-opener when we realized that lots of jobs could be performed from home, saving us money and time on travel and office rent. So far, so good. But there's a catch. Working from home greatly reduces daily mobility, which can create new, more toxic living conditions for a large part of society.

These new working conditions require new skills to help us maintain important components of physical and mental health. With the kitchen, its food cupboards, and the fridge, just a few steps away. Our work stations becoming another body part. And the lack of social interaction making face-to-face communication with important people in the working environment difficult or impossible.

It's a whole new ballgame. For all these reasons, working from home requires a lot of juggling every day. Are the people working from home aware of those new conditions, and the long-term challenges they represent?

And then there's AI, which takes all kinds of decisions for us; that's another set of challenges. It's true that the center of our health decision-making is moving further and further away. From the medications I need to take and their side effects, to the strange ingredients included in the products I eat every day; from the preventative surgeries that are suggested to me as I am a carrier of the X or Y gene, to the new miracle substance that removes fat and cellulite; from the biometric characteristics I share with the 'cloud' — that I don't know who else has access to — to the internet and social networks that make decisions about what I watch and consume daily.

It's so hard to know what to do about my health these days! It seems like the decisions I take are becoming more and more removed, and I feel gradually less empowered to take care of my health.

It would be helpful to know where and when I'm losing control over these decisions, and decide for my health status what I would like to do often (like what to do to increase my physical strength, which is connected to the health of my hormones and immune system) or less often (like what medication has the fewest side effects, and is most effective at reducing the discomfort in my throat).

The climate crisis is another reason that makes it tough to make the best decisions. The environment is changing, and it's becoming harder to maintain a healthy balance (relates to *homeostasis* which is the ability of the organism to maintain stable conditions inside (e.g., temperature, concentrations of various components) despite external changes in my functions).

With temperatures rising every year, we also frequently feel that we have a collective responsibility to act on climate change. And yes, it's important to have the right policies in place to reverse the climate crisis through the right policies, both at a state and an international level.

However, which are the right actions one can take at an individual level to help reverse climate change? It's quite simple. If each one of us could be more resilient and prepared (i.e. by being more fit and able to sustain extreme weather conditions), we could respond better to the abrupt environmental changes that climate change and its manifestations are putting us through.

I'd love to know if there's anything we can do as individuals to help reduce climate change and reverse climate crisis, contributing to real solutions. When it comes to individual responsibility, the need to prepare for climate change turns into a question of whether each person is preparing, through the right daily behaviors, to deal with it.

And if someone feels more vulnerable than they would like, is there anything they can do to strengthen personal resilience, and maintain optimism in the face of threat and impacts of climate change?

On a first level, reducing one's personal environmental footprint feels good. But separate from achieving that or not, how can each of us make our personal system physically and mentally stronger, so we can face climate challenges with the greatest resilience?

One thing is for sure: major climate changes require higher physical and mental capacities, which in turn help to maintain allostasis. Allostasis is a fancy word for the process of achieving stability or homeostasis in the body through continual physiological or behavioral changes. These changes required to function well could come from environmental alterations or adaptations in one's system. It's all about personal abilities.

As the demands of the environment we live in increase, it can be tough to prepare our systems optimally. Nevertheless, it's essential to be prepared, and it's great to see charities starting to issue relevant guidance to citizens. An Organization leading the way is www.americares.org, which emphasizes maximum preparation, readiness, and relief against climate change/disasters for citizens in many countries. Many other organizations are about to create similar directions, which is really encouraging.

The recent pandemic has shown us all just how important it is to be prepared; it's crucial to take care of one's body, mind, and spirit. By doing so, one gets the best chance of survival. For instance, being active and having better physical abilities has been, and still is, linked to improved chances of survival — but also great for one's health and quality of life.

Now, let me tell you a little bit about myself as a writer.

Why am I starting by writing a book about physical movement? It's important to remember that physical activity affects every single human system. From the way we express important genes in our biological mechanisms, to how we feel mentally and cognitively, and the ways we experience our relationships. It affects what and how much we eat, our cardiovascular, hormonal, respiratory, gastroesophageal, and immune systems, and the way our brain communicates with all other organs — especially the nervous and digestive systems. All of this makes physical movement the most central human behavior.

When one improves personal physical abilities, one is increasingly able to face various challenges in current society. For instance, one can endure cold or heat for longer, move with more ease, stand more upright, walk or run for longer, sleep better, and adapt to environmental demands successfully (through the maintenance of homeostatic and allostatic functions). This means that one can play a part in reducing the personal environmental footprint by making positive choices, and being an active, healthy, and engaged citizen.

It's necessary to take care of one's body, mind, and spirit every day. It's all about understanding one's own needs and turning awareness into a habit. This is where human society will meet its next challenges.

The information and suggestions in this book are based on solid scientific studies and are the result of years of research. Lots of helpful bibliographic references are included, for readers who would like to learn more about any research finding or pursue more information.

Our every decision is a product of personal choice and responsibility. Individual decisions affect not just us, but also our loved ones and others close to us, as well as those living nearby or far away. Similarly to the function of 'mirror neurons' in our brains (Bonini, et al., 2022), everyone's actions tend to imitate others', and influence others' actions, so, it's only natural that our personal choices affect the wider society — whether we realize it or not.

Let's share the love of science!

Enjoy this reading.

"With faith, with love, with our blood, that is, with human materials, the unparalleled is formed and the great leap from one civilization to the next, is made."

Nikos Kazantzakis, *"The Ascent"*

We and Our Loved Ones

It has been many years since my ancestors first started living with you, the human. You are such a wonderful creature, capable of great things! Ever since you first appeared on the planet, you've been amazing us with your ability to survive and thrive through invention and innovation. You've been able to harness fire, water, copper, and iron. You came to share your amazing existence with other living beings.

We belong to the Canidae family, which is part of the Carnivora tribe. We've been given the lovely name of 'domestic dogs'. This is in stark contrast to our wild counterparts who roam free. We're the first animals to live in your environment, right next to you, sharing your homes and living conditions. Of course, we're proud of that! No other mammal has been able to adapt to your sophisticated daily routine in the way we have. We've been living, working, and hunting alongside you for a very long time! That's why we've been by your side during the last 20,000 years of your evolutionary journey.

That is why I am dealing with you and your society, describing your habits and your living conditions. There is no one better suited to do this than I, a representative of the genus "Canis familiaris", since I have been an eyewitness to your daily life and your evolution. For more than 300,000 years you have been the most evolved mammal, the so-called "homo sapiens", the "wise man".

The very close and unique relationship we have developed together made me want to tell this story. Thousands of years of companionship, endless moments of togetherness. The bond we have developed is such that there is no other living being on Earth that can understand you better than we can. Imagine how many things we could share if we were able to speak your language.

Having lived in your house since I was very young, I spend all day with you and I can understand your joy and sadness, your excitement and enthusiasm. I admire you for many things.

I'll start with the organ that sets you apart from the rest of the creatures on Earth: your brain. You have a brain like ours, but it's much more sophisticated. You can communicate through complex concepts, provoking endless conversations. You have been able to develop your civilization, solving many problems that we consider unsolvable — or even unthinkable.

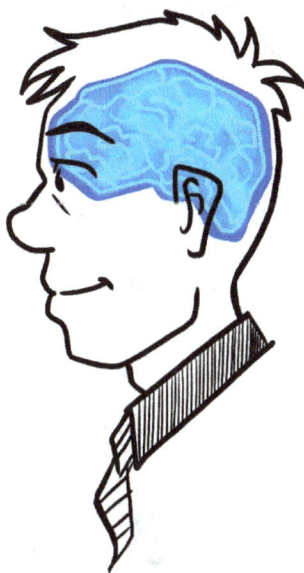

The Evolution

Your coveted evolution is one of the topics I would like to address. It has provided you with an abundance of comfort and convenience. Survival, in the richest and so-called evolved places of your environment, is easier than ever. Food is everywhere. Your travel is fast and easy. Your communication is approaching the speed of light.

And of course, energy. You spend more and more of it to keep this system running all the time. All kinds of energy. From chemical, which turns liquids into gases, to nuclear, which becomes heat and electricity. The problem with energy is that it's always going to be less than you need to continue to develop your civilization in the direction that it's going now. At least that is the case with your increasing population on Earth, and your fierce competition for global influence and profit with the rest of your species.

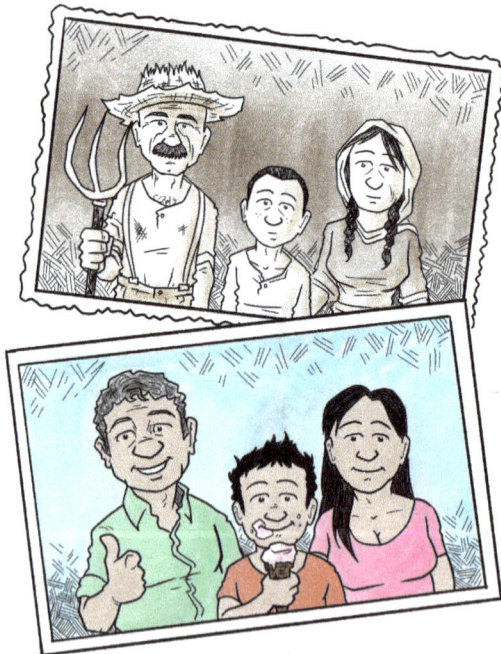

Only one kind of energy is so concentrated that it becomes excessive and overabundant. The more it is concentrated, the more it creates the conditions for crisis. And that crisis is too toxic to ignore.

The more excess energy you have, the more your body stores it. That's what we call stored fat. The more it accumulates, the more it hinders your quality of life and increases the likelihood of various metabolic diseases. Many things become more difficult. I know this about us dogs, as well. Often, we too become "victims" of this excess energy that is stored and which makes things difficult for us.

Although I understand a lot about you humans and can keep you very good company — better than any other beings on the planet — I still cannot understand many of your habits. When it comes to your body, soul, and spirit, you usually ignore your real needs, and you seem to have self-destructive tendencies. There's no other way to explain it, as you continue to hold on to many harmful habits that have a negative effect not only on you, but also on your family and the rest of your loved ones.

I also wonder why you don't use the most valuable thing you have in your life. It's a substance that is all around you. But you, the wise individual, are not receiving it. There are obviously many reasons for doing that, and I will try to explain them below. However, before doing that, it is better to start with the miraculous substance.

Imagine a substance that can heal every inflammation and physiological abnormality that may exist or develop in your body. At the same time, it strengthens your defenses against any type of invader. Its molecules are so potent that in a very short time, they provide substantial results by significantly improving your quality of life. This substance exists and can be one of the most important elixirs for preserving your youth.

Think of this substance as a lake next to the place we live and commute daily. Close to your work place. The lake is full of this magical substance, and you only need to step into its waters to receive its myriad benefits. Both we, the dogs, and you humans, are free to take a swim in it, every single day. The problem begins when you ignore the wonderful liquid of this lake. The more you ignore it, the harder it becomes to find where it is and to swim in its water. The more you avoid the lake, the more difficult it becomes to receive its miraculous benefits.

But if it is important to swim in its waters, how can you choose to ignore it? How can you, along with your wise human brain, make such a big mistake? How can you choose and continue to live away from the wondrous lake with its magical waters?

Unfortunately, it is in your nature to ignore the lake and its magical essence. Many of your habits associated with addictive substances, found in your every step, cause you to dislike the lake and its magical waters. These substances are the Trojan Horse of your body and mind: the more you use them, the more toxic they become. Similarly, the more frequently you rely on them, the more your brain needs them in your daily life. So, on the one hand, your body becomes more and more addicted to their presence, and on the other hand, the more you use them, the harder it becomes to swim or just splash around the Magic Lake.

The amazing thing is that you, who use those substances daily, already know how they work and how they may become toxic to your health. Yet, you continue to choose them. It takes a lot of effort and determination to stop using addictive substances.

These substances are everywhere and there are many of your species who rely on them. Let's take a better look at them.

The Substances

But which are these substances? You can find a lot of information about those in the following sentence: "Addiction is sweet and intoxicating in its smoke". In other words, the more you use these substances, the more you increase your need to use them repeatedly and in increasing amounts.

Sugar, alcohol, and nicotine are the three most common addictive substances for you and your species. And, of course, they are the main causes of your withdrawal from the miracle lake, as they make it difficult to have regular contact with it. Their use also creates multiple problems in your system, accelerating the ageing of your tissues and significantly reducing your quality of life.

Sugar meets your body and brain's energy needs in the short and medium term (for the next three to five hours of your day). For thousands of years, you found this energy in fruits and vegetables. But since you discovered sugar and its easy production, this energy is easily provided by foods you and other humans create and contain it in abundance.

Unfortunately, the food industry you created has made sure that sugar is everywhere: in bread, ketchup, grains, and convenience food. The ease of preserving industrially produced foods (sugary products are toxic to any other organisms, so they become resistant to bacteria, as well) and the need to increase sales (preference for these foods over other competing food types) have put sugar in almost all the industrialized types of food you produce in large quantities (e.g. carbonated beverages). The problem is that the consumptio of such an increased amount of sugar has become a central source of energy for you, and you unconsciously choose foods that contain it avoiding the "tasteless" foods that don't contain added sugar (e.g. vegetables). You have come to overly favor industrialized over natural foods.

Natural food types like fruits give your body enough energy without raising blood sugar levels, as they combine the right amount of sweetness and insoluble fiber. This happens as natural, non-industrialized food types create a lower absorption of sugars, causing less insulin secretion from the pancreas and significantly reducing sugar spikes in your blood stream.

The opposite happens when you frequently consume industrialized food types and a high level of added sugars. Absorbing those puts your metabolism at risk. These mass-produced foods and beverages that contain high amounts of sugar — but also other sugar alternatives, such as high fructose corn syrup and / or other sweeteners such as aspartame, which has many unpleasant health effects since your system does not recognize it — cause you to secrete more insulin, gain fat, and put on body weight by adding 'empty calories' lacking any significant nutritional elements (i.e. vitamins).

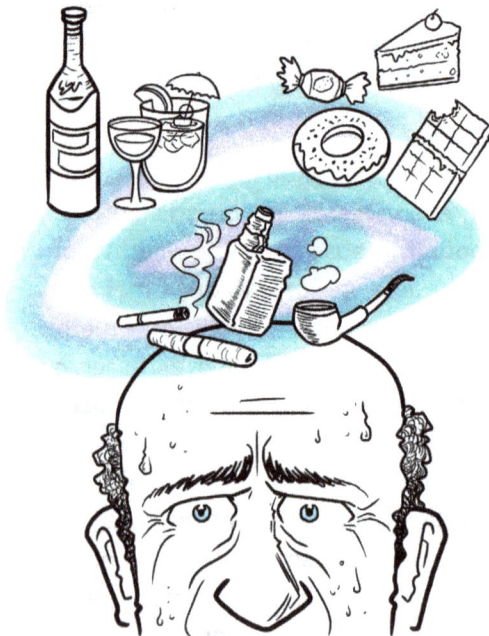

Since increased sugar consumption begins at an early age, the addiction of the younger generation of your species is even greater. Diseases directly related to sugar consumption have become increasingly common in recent decades. This toxic habit has become almost synonymous with chronic health problems such as diabetes mellitus, cognitive decline and, of course, obesity. Sugar's addictive nature means your body finds it difficult to take the plunge into the miracle lake, because your systems of transporting and consuming energy are alienated and cannot cope with the demands of the miracle substance. This alienation can take the form of metabolic diseases that you and your species suffer from. These include pre-diabetes, metabolic syndrome, cardiovascular disease, hypertension, triglycerides, etc.

Nicotine and the addiction caused by smoking is another habit that makes it difficult to receive the miracle substance. The reason here relates to the difficulty of your body to take in oxygen. The longer you smoke over a lifetime, the more you reduce the oxygen levels that reach your body and tissues, and the harder it is for your body to function properly to perform its daily movements. It becomes increasingly difficult to perform activities such as running, walking, avoiding obstacles, and climbing stairs. It is no coincidence that most regular smokers avoid these activities.

Hence, if you smoke regularly, the harder it is for your system to move, and you will increasingly choose to avoid moving or using your body. This leads to a kind of motor disability, starting with seemingly unnecessary movements in everyday life (e.g. walking or climbing stairs) and progressing to avoidance of bodily activities and increased sedentariness. It comes as a normal consequence that the less you move your system, the higher the difficulty is to get to the lake and enjoy the benefits of its wondrous waters.

Alcohol is another agent that makes it difficult for your body to reach the miracle lake. It provides 'empty calories' that increase your body fat, fatiguing your vital organs (e.g. liver and kidneys), and reducing your muscles' ability to function, grow, and continue operating.

These three substances trick your system and cause increasing damage to your body through their addictive effects. Unfortunately, your "smart" system, that evolved through processes of hundreds of thousands of years, chooses them more over time. Their immediate effects deceive your system and as a result you increase their consumption.

What is even more unfortunate is that this triad has managed to infiltrate your society for good and has become identified with feelings of comfort and relaxation. Thus, these substances — along with others I will discuss next — become increasingly popular, they are chosen by numerous of your kind, and they cause a multitude of diseases. Sadly, addictions created by those three substances lead to significant illnesses, with many of your species forced to moderate their intake before it is too late.

Luckily, there is a way to remove those three substances from your life. Firstly, you need to be willing to improve your health. This has to do with what you perceive you may gain or lose by getting rid of these substances.

Based on what I've seen, appreciating that regular consumption of these substances is linked to sickness, makes you want to change what you're doing. When you understand their toxic effects, you tend to change. Simply and swiftly.

On a second level, it relates to whether and how much you feel able to change. This relates to your motives and what makes your behavior more effective. More about this in the following chapters. All I can mention here is that by choosing to change, you can reduce their effects right away. It just takes determination and self-control.

Unfortunately, when you and your species are addicted, you

don't like to change. I understand that, as I love you and I have seen how you react to them. However, it never ceases to upset me observing you, the wise and intelligent human, destroying yourself through your addictions. And most importantly, to see that through your addictions, you move even further from the Magic Lake and its miraculous liquid.

For example, when consuming these substances frequently, you are in greater need of them, and you are entering into the habit of using them in increased volumes. Habits are not easy to change. Especially when you have no indication that your body is being harmed by consuming such substances.

Another great benefit of the Magic Lake is that the more you use it, the more you understand what's good and bad for you. Using the Lake's waters makes your system increasingly sensitive to small changes occurring in daily living, making you feel either better or worse. You are in a position to protect yourself better, since it is easier to appreciate how you respond to the substances of your environment —before they cause further damage. Another reason I am calling the Lake, a Magic one!

I also realized that in addition to these substances, there are other things in your environment that can become addictive, making the visit to the Lake and its magical essence difficult. For example, you may be over-consumed with your job, or the screens you are staring at for hours. Without a conscious effort, they tend to sabotage or alienate you from your fellow humans, and deter you from using the waters of the Magic Lake.

Coming back to the magic substance, I have noticed that one of its key features relates to children: children and infants of your species receive the substance generously and without much effort. When left free, they find and receive the magic elements of the Lake through an innate instinct, without conscious effort. And when in a position to explore the Magic Lake daily, it provides excellent results for their development, laying the best foundations for their long-term health.

But enough about what causes the aversion of the Magic Lake and its element. Better to talk about its ingredients. It consists of—

Now that I think about it, it's too early to reveal its ingredients. Let me save them for later, for I risk losing the essence of my story. If I reveal the substance, it is very likely you will stop reading the story and just go out and try to buy it. I'm afraid it is not that easy to find it, though.

I will lighten your impatience by revealing some of its key features. One important feature of the magic substance is that if you stop taking it for any reason, you must reintroduce it gradually and carefully. Otherwise, it can cause some sort of allergy and unwanted side effects. Reduced dose or deviation from the substance must be treated seriously and with the help of a specialist. This is the only way to avoid the manifestation of an allergy to the magical substance, which is associated with high toxicity and a decline in quality of life.

A major problem is that although many of your species know about the benefits of the miracle substance, very few of them use it in daily living. It seems that the more you know about the benefits of this substance, the less of your kind take advantage of its positive effects and miraculous particles.

The good thing is that those of your species already familiarized with the miraculous Lake, talk often about their habit of diving into its waters and receiving its valuable properties. However — and quite surprisingly — the more they talk, the less those who refuse to acknowledge the Lake want to know about it! It never ceases to amaze me, no matter how many times I see it.

One of the root causes of the problem is the continuous determination required to be in a position to receive the positive effects of this substance; it takes constant effort and commitment to explore its components. A day, a week, or a month of exploration is not enough. This fact reveals another paradox of the Magic Lake: those already using it suggest they can't do without it. But for the rest, it is not a necessity. They simply live their lives without it, choosing to ignore it.

It is clear, then, that the Magic Lake requires energy and constant exploration for its components to be discovered. It is offered to those of your species who have the energy to systematically seek it out, and to explore the ways they can receive its effects.

Likewise, as the age of the Lake seeker increases, its substance becomes more challenging to explore. The reason is simple: the later one finds it, the more difficult it gets to familiarize oneself with its constant use. This results in an increased distance between those familiar with its magical elements and the rest who haven't discovered it. Similarly, the further the body gets from its normal propensities and the potential to discover its rejuvenating elements, the harder the finding of this matter tends to be.

For the above reasons, those who try to promote the miraculous substance to you humans do not have an easy time. Non-users of the Lake find influencers odd, others find them slow-witted. What is certain is that those of you who use the Magic Lake and its empowering essence live better, have more control over their lives, and are happier with their choices. They have a better quality of life, which is associated with fewer health problems, higher self-esteem, more confidence in the present, and greater optimism for the future.

The good news is that no matter how far you and your species have strayed from the Magic Lake, there is always the prospect of discovering it. If you pursue it enough and are determined to find it, you will be able to harvest its advantages. In doing so, former toxic impulses or habits will fade, and you will reap the maximum benefit from its miraculous substance.

The Stroll

I go crazy with joy every time they open the door for me to go out for my walk. I jump from chair to chair, I run from right to left, I try to pull on my leash. It's the joy of my day.

My caretakers often resent me. They argue about whose turn it is to take me out. They don't seem to be very eager to go out for a second time and do the same thing. The beginning of their stroll with me is always difficult, the first steps are tentative and indecisive. And when the weather is wintry, the difficulty is even greater. At least in the beginning.

After the first steps, my minder follows without objection. It's like something magical is initiating. I sniff ahead, eager to move on to the next scent. They — that is, whoever I convince to walk with me — follow my movements with interest. When I finally stop to begin the defecating process, I can tell by their movements and tugging on the leash whether they are allowed to do so or not.

It is the need to leave my tracks and to smell the pheromones of the other dog friends who hang out in the neighborhood. Not all are appealing; I'm interested in leaving my tracks to define my territory. You never know when the next friend will walk by, smell, and remember me the next time we're together. And then ... let the games begin!

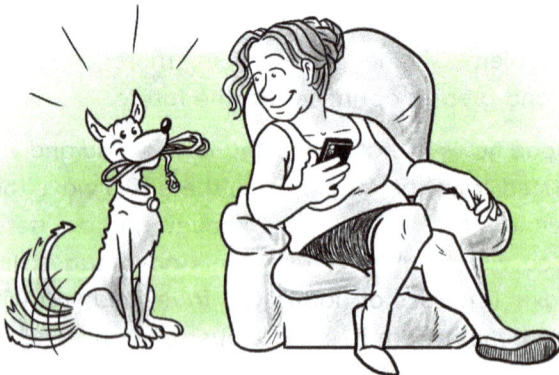

But back to my caretakers and their friends. Thank God they have me. I wag my tail and remind them of my walk time. They can just sit in the chair for hours without even realizing it. They often have their attention focused on a big, square screen in front of them that keeps showing stories, with pictures and sounds. *Lots* of pictures and *lots* of sounds. It changes all the time, and I think that's very attractive to their eyes. They don't take their eyes off it for hours!

Other times they sit in front of a smaller screen. They have a different posture, their hands are right under the screen, and they hit some black shapes for hours. Or they talk to the screen. Strange things.

They obviously find something amusing there. From what I hear, the problem is that they sit for hours and hours without getting up, even for a few minutes. If they chose to stand up for just five minutes every hour, their bodies would be able to keep their metabolism active. What happens during the time they are sitting or lying down (some choose to do that while looking at their screens) is toxic to their system: basic metabolic processes stop, and along with the brain, all their organs go into "safe mode". They simply exist, using less and less energy.

It is not only the sitting position, but also what they choose to do when they are in that position. The big screen is the biggest problem. The countless hours spent there cause the most harm, as they are completely passive. They just watch images passing by. Without making any kind of effort to change what they see. And even if they do try to change something, it is at the touch of a button so they do not need to make any effort or go near the big, square screen.

It was not like that before. If you wanted to change any images and sounds, you had to go next to the square screen — it was a square box back then — and press a button. You had to move around a lot, so the big screen was less of a problem than it currently is. Until an inventor produced the idea of restricting your movements even more. It was 1955 when a Zenith engineer, Eugene Polley (1915-2012), built a box — he called it the Flash-matic — that could interfere with the stories on the screen without you and your friends having to get up from your seats. For over 50 years, you and your species thought you owed him a favor. But then you realized that the screen you are seeing these stories on, and Polley's box, were hurting you. Very badly. These two in conjunction are so bad that they can cause chronic pain, disease, and even shorten your life span!

Yes, you read that right. The more passive you and your species become to the stories and sounds of the screen, and the more time you spend in front of the screen each day, the more likely you are to get sick and shorten your life span. In fact, those in the know say that every hour you go without getting off the couch, things get increasingly serious. And when you reach or exceed four hours in front of the big screen, it is even more certain that you are harming your health (Park et al., 2020; Saunders, McIsaac, Douillette, et al., 2020).

Fortunately, you have me and my other four-legged friends to keep you moving, as long as you take us for walks. On the other hand, there are other things you can do while sitting that aren't so bad for you. For example, sitting while eating, talking to others, or watching a small screen is much better. This is because you spend less time sitting, or because you are keeping your brain more active while you do these things.

From what I hear, not all sedentary (being seated position for a long time, while being physically inactive) activities have the same negative effects. This happens as on one hand they are more frequently interrupted (e.g. reading a book), and on the other, they do not attract your attention as effectively through captivating lights and sounds.

Most importantly, any sedentary pursuit that does not involve a big screen full of sounds and stories makes you more alert, actively involved in what is going on around you, activating all your organs — including your brain. This is why, with all the other activities you spend in a sitting position, the problem starts when you are sedentary for more than seven hours a day — and gets worse when you sit for more than eight hours a day (Park et al., 2020).

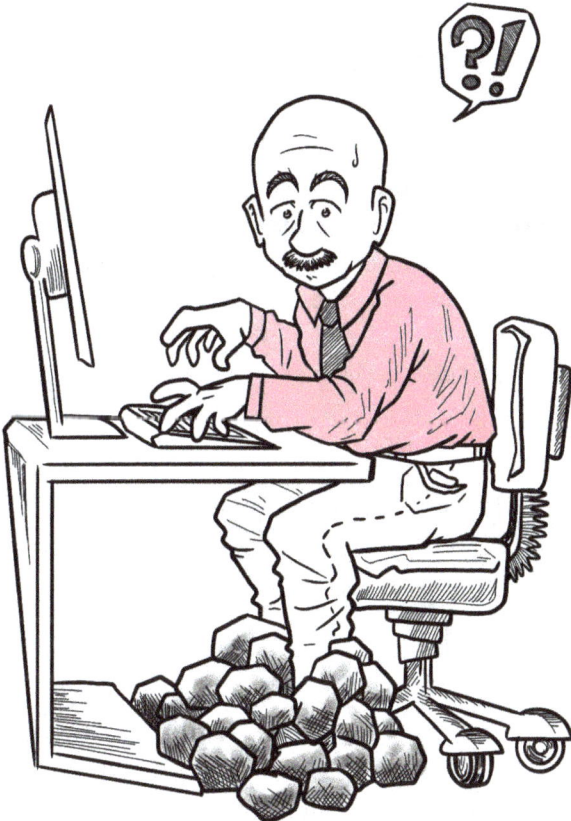

For all these reasons, you should often remember how much you owe us and how grateful you humans should be to us and our breeds. Those who know, say that the more you walk with us the less toxic your harmful habits become. More precisely, if you manage to walk with us for more than an hour per day, you tend to reduce the risk of harm and injury, protecting your health by more than 30% (Wohlrab, Klenk, Delgado-Ortiz, 2022).

Nice and simple, don't you think? Walking with us for an hour a day will not only improve your physical health, but also your mental health. Walking will help you escape from your worries, fears, and stress. That is, if you do not look at the screen that you usually have in your hand or, even better, if you leave your phone at home.

Hence, it is time to adopt one of my species if you have not done it already. Every time you take a walk with your four-legged friend, you will feel more energized and refreshed on all levels. I am sure, your mental and physical health will be greatly improved!

The Magic Lake

Swimming in the sea is a real pleasure. Even for us dogs. On sizzling summer days, I do not want to get out of the water. If you don't play fetch with me, I will stay in the water all day long!

Now imagine that you are swimming in magical waters. Imagine that every time you dive into them, they make you a better person. In every way. On every level. In all functions. Every minute you spend in these magical waters, every single organ — every cell in your body — is in better working condition.

These magical waters are the remedy for every condition. Every ailment. It is the existing substance that heals every health problem.

If you knew that a drug or a pill could cure your every malfunction, make you feel better where you need it most, how much money would you give to get it? Obviously, a lot of your savings. If I told you it is more expensive than that, how much would you save to try to get it?

It is indeed expensive. But it cannot be bought with money. It requires love and care instead. And increased enthusiasm, every single day. But also, a steady investment of time.

Oh, I should not forget trust. Trust in your ability to improve. But also, in your potential to turn constant effort into habit. And when you manage to create this habit, you can receive the substance generously and without delay.

In short, the Magic Lake and its waters are about your mood, your motivation, and an hour in your day. It is also as cheap as the air you breathe and the energy you spend.

If all these confuse you, but at the same time make you want to explore the Magic Lake further, you are on the right track. Trust me, every minute you spend exploring the lake and its secrets is worth it! All these relate to you, your explorations, and your accomplishments. No intermediary is required and there is no need for anyone to prepare the essence of the Magic Lake for you.

Every time you command your body to move, you are on the right track; in the direction of the magical waters of the lake. Over 600 biochemical factories are ready to produce the magic ingredient that will make you feel better in no time. Just as long as it takes for the magic substance to reach every cell, organ, and center of your system. That is — immediately!

It's time to reveal the big secret: what the Magic Lake is, where you can find it, and how to swim in its elements, acquiring all its magical qualities.

It's a substance you can find through physical movement. Every move you make benefits your system in a unique way. And the benefits are magically multiplied as every movement follows the next. With every inch of its surface and every foot you travel across it, the Magic Lake holds numerous surprises for you to explore.

It's no exaggeration to mention that every moment you choose to swim in its magical waters, the benefits to your body increase geometrically, and you gradually become the jaguar you've always wanted. And the best part is that, under the right conditions, the whole experience is such a pleasure that it can replace many of your not-so-healthy habits.

For example, smoking. The more you move, the less inclined your lungs are to taste the tar and nicotine in cigarettes (Hassandra, Goudas, and Theodorakis, 2015). The reasons are many. For one, the body and its energy-producing systems are already busy generating energy for you to keep moving. They have neither the time nor the inclination to add substances that interfere with these processes.

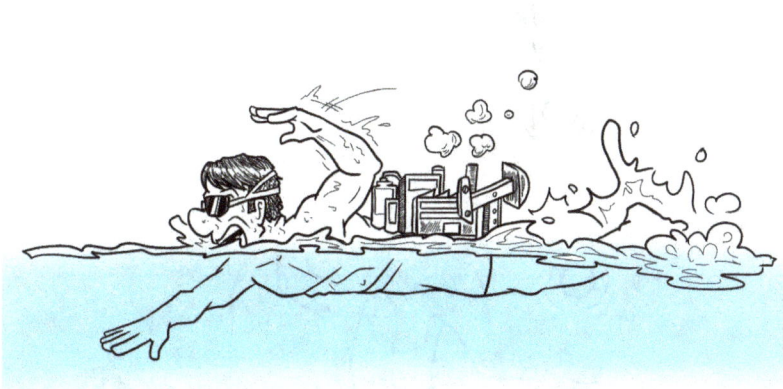

On the other hand, the brain is interested in other forms of neurotransmitters (serotonin, dopamine, etc.; neurotransmitters are chemical compounds used to pass important-critical life-continuity information from one brain neuron — or cell — to the next, or to a muscle neuron to produce movement, or to a gland for hormone production) which are released in abundance during exercise. The tendency to light a cigarette decreases as the satisfaction from frequent physical movement and exercise increases. It's as simple as that.

I agree, this is not enough to change your habits. In fact, it is too early to make such decisions. Let's first address the reasons that make the lake magical. There are so many — too many to ignore.

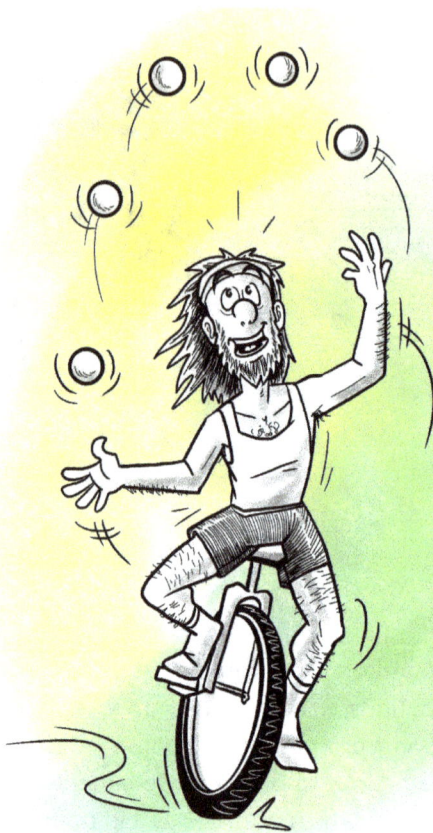

First of all, every metric related to health improves with a simple 20 or 30 minutes of physical activity. It improves even more after a period of one, three, or six months of regular physical activity participation. Most importantly, such physical activity does not have to be intense. Simple and repetitive movements performed without panting (i.e., low or moderate intensity, in the language of those introduced to the exercise terms) are enough to start and continue this chain of beneficial effects on every cell and organ in your system. There are numerous studies confirming these positive effects, each time assessing the impact of physical activity on thousands of participants like you.

For example, proteomic analysis (proteomic analysis or proteomics refers to the systematic identification and quantification of the entire complement of proteins, the proteome, of a biological system -cell, tissue, organ, biological fluid, or organism- at a given time), shows that some of the most basic cellular functions which indicate good health are inextricably attached to exercise. Factors such as liver fat, kidney filtration capacity, percentage of body fat, visceral fat mass, lean mass, cardiovascular function, alcohol consumption, smoking, and cardiovascular risk are associated with physical activity and its effects (Ahadi et al., 2020).

How, for example, can physical activity be the solution to alcohol consumption? Quite simply, the toxicity of alcohol prevents cells from functioning. In other words, when your system goes through the process of performing repetitive physical movements, the transfer of energy, oxygen, and all other changes occurring to support these processes send a message to your brain's decision centers — hypothalamus, thalamus, and frontal lobes — that alcohol and its effects are not allowing the body to function well. It's that simple. Through regular physical activity, your system becomes "allergic" to what disturbs and reduces its capabilities.

Dopamine

Dopamine is one of the neurotransmitters in your brain. It acts as a messenger, a chemical released by neurons (nerve cells) to send signals to other nerve cells. Neurotransmitters are synthesized in specific areas of the brain and systematically affect many areas of your behavior and decision-making.

For example, the brain contains several different dopamine pathways, one of which plays an important role in motivating your reward-driven behavior. Anticipating reward increases dopamine levels in your brain.

Various addictive substances increase the release of dopamine, or block its reuptake into your neurons after it is released. Dopamine is also involved in motor control and the release of various hormones. It is precisely this mechanism that is responsible for various changes that occur in the nervous system because of your behavior and choices.

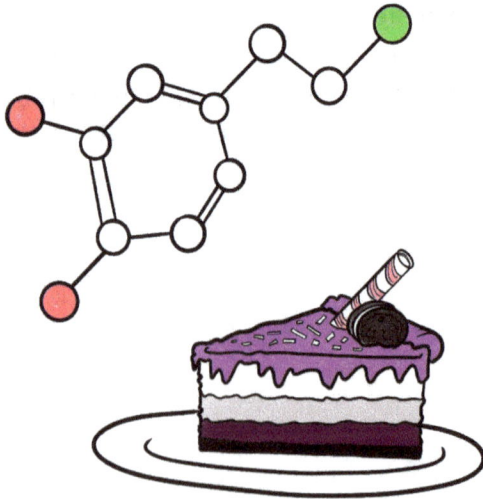

According to neuroscience, dopamine is considered one of the pleasure chemicals. It is directly linked to the reward systems that mediate the brain's responses to so-called opioids (also known as natural or synthetic drugs), i.e., food or other pleasurable stimuli and images that you see every day.

Think about how your brain reacts when you're in front of your favorite treat. Is it chocolate or cream? Sweet or savory? It doesn't really matter to your pleasure detection and tracking system. Your previous positive experience is enough for this system to try to repeat that action.

Hence, you don't focus on anything other than the expected taste and pleasure. The moment you taste that delicacy again. During the moment of anticipation, there is nothing else in the world. You are simply focusing on the treat that is about to meet your tongue and palate, releasing its taste and texture.

It is that moment your brain synchronizes with its dopaminergic response, with many brain cells releasing the dopamine neurotransmitter. The way you experience this explains its power: your mood improves, you're available for social interactions, your system gets into a positive mood, and you feel ready for the rest of the day.

A key effect of the Magic Lake is related to this very neurotransmitter, dopamine. Simply put, regular physical activity improves your mood, and sets the stage for intensified productivity and efficiency throughout the day.

Avoiding the Magic Lake

The opposite happens to the brain and its neurotransmitters when you experience negative events, which have an impact on the way you perceive yourself and your environment. Your body then tries to avoid such negative events.

That's where the problem lies: frequent avoidance of such events leads to permanent changes in your behavior, as the fear of them increases, a direct result of which is an even stronger propensity to keep away from similar events in the future. And when these adverse experiences lead to chronic or intense reactions, they can contribute to the development of severe psychological responses or even stress-related psychiatric disorders, such as post-traumatic stress disorder, generalized anxiety, or even depression.

But what happens when kinetic activities are associated with distress and negative experiences from an early age?

Negative comments from teachers and peers, comparisons with the physical performance of others, perhaps even mocking comments about one's appearance, make up a series of experiences that sooner or later lead to keeping away from various forms of physical activity. If this happens at an early age, it will shape one's future choices.

Unfortunately, negative experiences from such previous incidents do cause avoidance of physical activity; in these cases, engaging the body in any kind of movement automatically causes intolerance. No matter what experts may suggest and how helpful towards keeping active one's social and physical environment may be. Any opportunities for being active, or recommendations for increased participation in exercise programs to improve health, tend to be ignored. Denial is the most common response to such exhortations, wherever they come from.

This is exactly where frequent and varied positive experiences of physical activity are needed to reverse this experience. What does this mean?

It simply means that you provide yourself every opportunity to move, while having fun. In ways that make your movements easy and pleasant. For as comfortably or as long you want your movement to be.

The good news is that when you engage frequently in an enjoyable form of physical activity, it can soon become a habit. No matter how short this bout of physical activity may be, it can significantly reduce the adverse effects of previous negative physical activity experiences. This is effective and has an increasingly positive effect on your decision-making system.

Over the past three decades, many studies have shown that regular participation in physical activity improves mental and physical health, and allows you to be more resilient and tolerant in demanding everyday circumstances. In the long term, this leads to better emotional control, self-efficacy, confidence, and satisfaction with daily activities. And over time, a better quality of life.

In addition to reducing the incidence of mental health disorders, frequent exercise reduces anxiety responses and the sensitivity of the psychophysiological axis of anxiety and catecholamine (e.g., adrenaline) release. Consequently, regular physical activity participation leads to increased optimism and expectations of positive outcomes in daily endeavors, even in patients with chronic depression (Dishman, 1997; Crush, Frith, and Loprinzi, 2018).

Let me be clearer.

At any given point, your system comprehends having a certain level of fitness. For example, you can run continuously and at a certain speed for 17 minutes, not for 20 minutes. You can bench press 50kgs, not 60kgs. You can run as fast as you can for 40 meters, not 80. These performances depend on how often, for how long, and what type of activities you do each day, week, or month. These are the activities that determine how your system perceives and translates your experience each time you choose to move.

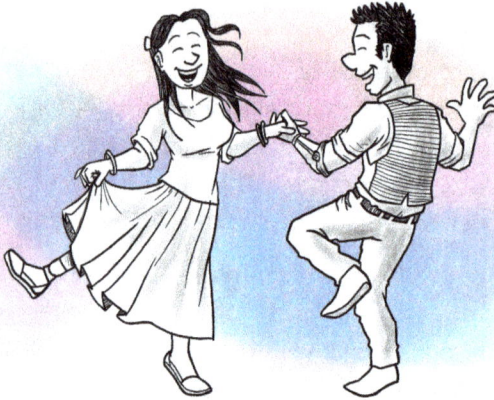

Let me remind you again of dopamine and how it is released every time you eat your favorite treat. How is that experience different from the way the brain reacts when you are about to move or when you are moving?

What kind of feeling do you have every time you do some kind of kinetic activity?

Ideally, it's not much different than your reaction to your favorite dessert. But to do that, you need to appreciate your fitness level (in terms of strength, endurance, speed, and flexibility), how your body feels, and how you experience your quality of life in the present moment.

It sounds complicated, but it's not. All you need to do is choose to engage in a physical activity that you like, for as long as you continue to enjoy doing so. When your experience begins to change, you simply stop. Taking note of the duration of the motor activity, along with its other elements (e.g., was it brisk walking or light running? Was it uphill, straight road, or downhill?) will give you enough information about your current physical condition.

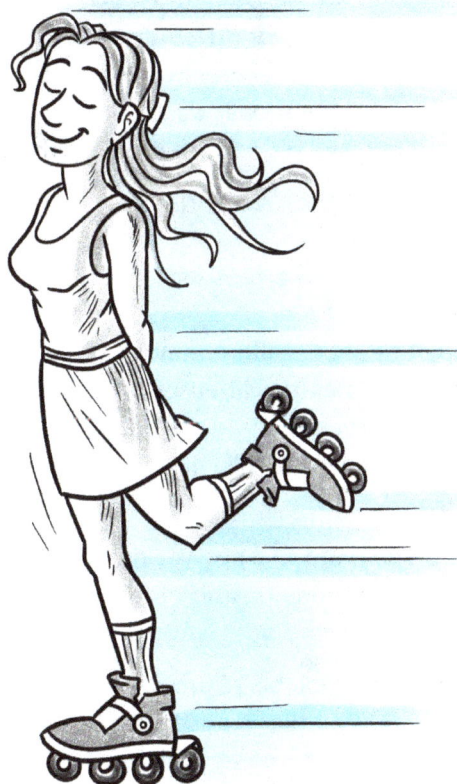

What does your brain, and the dopamine it releases, suggest about this experience? Given that you continue to perform the exercise you enjoy as frequently as you like, soon you will be able to undertake your preferred activities for longer. This will enhance your fitness levels and enable you to engage in your preferred activity with greater ease and enjoyment.

Repetition and improved endurance lead to enhanced ease of movement and greater enjoyment. They also lead to improvements in key indicators of physical and mental health. And, consequently, to a higher quality of life.

How Much Exercise Do You Need?

I do know that the World Health Organization (WHO) guidelines and recommendations provide details for different age groups and specific populations, as to how much physical activity is needed to achieve a good level of health for your species.

Specifically, the World Health Organization (WHO, 2020) recommends that:

For children under 5

In a 24-hour period, **children under 12 months** should be physically active several times in a variety of ways, especially through interactive play on the ground. The more the better, and always within the normal limits that each child perceives adequate (without pressure to move more).

For infants who are not yet mobile, this includes at least 30 minutes in the prone position (on their stomach or face down on the floor) during the day, while they are awake.

They should not be restrained for more than one hour at a time (e.g., in a stroller / pushchair, highchair, or strapped to the back of the parent / caregiver).

Also, no screen time is advised.

When appropriate, parent / caregiver involvement in reading and storytelling is encouraged. Combined with 14-17 hours (0-3 months) or 12-16 hours (4-11 months) of good quality sleep, including naps.

In a 24-hour period, **children of 1-2 years of age**, should:
Get at least 180 minutes of different types of physical activity of any intensity, including moderate to vigorous physical activity, spread throughout the day. The more physical activity, the better, but always within the normal limits that each child perceives adequate (without pressure to move more).

Children should not be restrained for more than one hour at a time (e.g., in a stroller / pushchair, highchair, or strapped to the back of a parent or caregiver) or be seated for long periods of time.

Sedentary screen time (e.g. watching TV or videos, playing computer games, etc.) is not recommended for children as young as one year of age.

Sitting in front of a computer screen or TV should not exceed one hour for children two years of age. The less sitting time, the better.

When children of this age are sedentary, it is good to encourage reading and storytelling by parents and caregivers, to help develop their imagination.

It is important that they get 11-14 hours of good quality sleep, including naps. Children of this age group should not exceed these normal sleeping and waking times.

In a 24-hour period, **children aged 3-4 years** should:
Spend at least 180 minutes in a variety of physical activities of all intensities, including at least 60 minutes of moderate or vigorous physical activity, spread throughout the day. The more physical activity, the better, but always within the limits of what each child feels is normal (no pressure to move more).

Children of that age group should not be sedentary (e.g. sitting) for more than one hour at a time (e.g. in a stroller / wheelchair) or for long periods of time (e.g. two, three or more hours).

Sitting in front of a computer screen or TV should not exceed one hour for 3-4-year-olds. The less sitting time, the better.

When sitting, it is important to engage in reading and storytelling with the parent or caregiver.

It is important to get 10-13 hours of good quality sleep, including short naps.

Children of this age group should not exceed these normal sleeping and waking times.

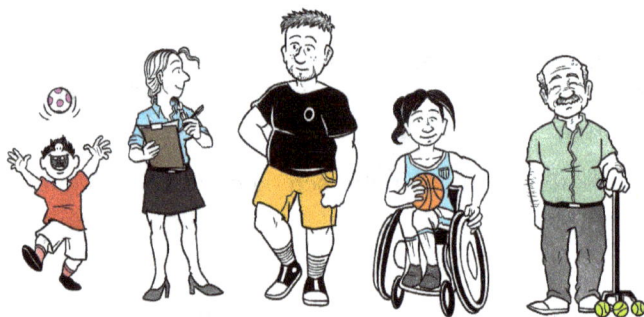

Children and adolescents aged 5-17 years;
Should get an average of at least 60 minutes of moderate-to-vigorous physical activity, mostly aerobic, each day during the week. (Intensity refers to how hard the system of an individual is working during exercise. During moderate intensity, the individual can still talk comfortably. However, during vigorous intensity – the individual is breathing hard and can only say a few words without pausing. Finally, high intensity activity refers to giving 100% of effort during a short period of time).

From 5 -17 years children and adolescents should include high-intensity aerobic activity and physical activity that strengthens muscles and bones, at least three days a week.

Children and adolescents of this age group should limit the amount of time they spend sedentary, and especially the amount of time they spend in front of a screen.

Adults aged 18-64;
Need at least 150-300 minutes of moderate intensity aerobic physical activity, or 75-150 minutes of higher intensity aerobic physical activity (or a similar combination of moderate and vigorous intensity physical activity), over the week.

For additional and important health benefits, adults of this age group also need to do moderate-to-vigorous intensity muscle-strengthening activities, involving all major muscle groups, two or more days a week.

This population category can increase moderate intensity aerobic activity to more than 300 minutes, or vigorous intensity aerobic activity to more than 150 minutes. Similarly, doing a combination of moderate and vigorous activity throughout the week can provide additional health benefits.

Adult populations of this category need to limit the amount of time spent sedentary. Replacing sedentary time with physical activity of any intensity (even low-intensity) provides significant health benefits.

To reduce the harmful health effects of a prolonged sedentary lifestyle it is imperative for all adults up till the age of 65 to try to get at least 150 minutes of moderate physical activity or 75 minutes of vigorous physical activity per week.

Adults of age 65 and older;
Need to follow the same guidelines as 18-64-year-olds.

During each week, seniors should engage in moderate- or vigorous-intensity physical activity that emphasizes functional balance and strengthening. Such programs are crucial for the maintenance of physical function, and need to be performed three or more days per week to improve functional capacity and prevent falls.

Pregnant and postpartum women;
Pregnant women and new mothers who have recently given birth — in the absence of medical contraindications — are recommended to choose a variety of aerobic and muscle-strengthening activities.

They also need to reduce time spent sedentary. Replacing sedentary time with a variety of physical activities of all intensities provides many health benefits.

People living with chronic health conditions (high blood pressure, type two diabetes, HIV, and former cancer patients);
Get at least 150-300 minutes of moderate-intensity, or 75-150 minutes of high-intensity, aerobic activity each week. Similarly, an equivalent combination of moderate- and vigorous-intensity activity is recommended over the week.

This population category also needs to do moderate-to-vigorous intensity muscle strengthening activities, that involve all major muscle groups, two or more days a week, as these provide significant health benefits.

As part of their weekly physical activity, older people living with health conditions need to engage in a variety of physical activities that emphasize functional balance and muscle-strengthening activities, of moderate or higher intensity, three or more days a week, to improve functional capacity and prevent falls.

They can also increase moderate intensity aerobic physical activity to more than 300 minutes, or do more than 150 minutes of vigorous intensity aerobic physical activity (or an equivalent combination of moderate and vigorous activity), throughout the week for additional health benefits.

Limit the time spent in sedentary activities, especially passive types of sedentary behaviors (i.e. TV watching), and replacing sedentary time with physical activity of any intensity, as it provides significant health benefits.

To reduce the adverse health effects of a sedentary lifestyle, all adults and older people are encouraged to aim for more than the recommended levels of moderate-to-vigorous physical activity.

Children and teens with disabilities;
Need to get an average of at least 60 minutes of moderate-to-vigorous physical activity, mostly aerobic, per week.

At least three days a week, they need to include high-intensity aerobic activity. They also need to include activities that strengthen muscles and bones.

Limit sedentary time, especially time spent watching TV or using a computer screen.

Adults who live with a disability;
Get at least 150-300 minutes of moderate intensity aerobic activity, 75-150 minutes of vigorous intensity aerobic activity, or an equivalent combination of moderate- and vigorous-intensity activity each week.

There is also a need to do moderate- or high-intensity muscle strengthening activities that use all major muscle groups two or more days a week, as these provide additional and important health benefits.

Older people with disabilities;
As part of their weekly physical activity, older people with disabilities need to engage in a program of varied physical activity that emphasizes functional balance and strengthening at moderate or higher intensity, three or more days per week, to improve functional capacity and prevent falls.

They can increase the duration of moderate intensity aerobic activity to more than 300 minutes or increase the duration of vigorous-intensity aerobic activity to more than 150 minutes. Alternatively, they are encouraged to perform a combination of moderate and vigorous activity most days of the week for additional health benefits.

There is a need to limit time spent in sedentary activities, especially passive forms of sedentariness (i.e. TV watching). There are significant health benefits in replacing sedentary time with physical activity of any intensity (even low intensity).

To reduce the adverse health effects of long periods of sedentary time, all adults and older people need to aim to exceed the recommended levels of moderate to vigorous physical activity.

There is also a need to avoid prolonged sitting. It is recommended to be physically active while sitting or lying down. For example, perform upper body activities, sports, and activities if there is a need to use regularly special equipment or a wheel chair.

For more information:
World Health Organization. guidelines on physical activity and sedentary behavior. Geneva: World Health Organization; 2020.

You may download the World Health Organization guidelines by scanning this pictogram.

Reduced Physical Activity

All of the previous guidelines are provided by the World Health Organization, because of the reduced participation in physical activity that you and your species are engaging with. Sadly, as far as I know, decreased participation in physical activity during the last thirty years has reached a pandemic level.

Societies that show reduced participation in physical activity are more prone to disease and premature death. This has now been thoroughly demonstrated by numerous epidemiological studies (e.g. de Souto Barreto, 2013). Reduced physical activity (relative to the recommended levels of physical activity) is the 4th most common cause of premature death, and one of the leading causes of physical and mental illness in modern societies.

Unfortunately, this is despite the wealth of information on the importance of regular physical activity for good health and quality of life. But what is causing the decline in physical activity participation? Does the reduced response to these messages reflect a refusal to accept scientific evidence? A closer look helps explain the problem.

First, regular physical activity competes with your modern lifestyle. Your sense of time has changed. After a working day spent in front of a computer screen, you quite often rush home to spend additional time in front of the TV. Whatever time you gain by using motorized transportation, you tend to spend it watching a screen again: a mobile phone or personal computer for social networking and computer games, or a TV for watching your favorite shows.

But the modern lifestyle also affects your sense of physical movement. The things that you used to do twenty or thirty years ago, before many of your movements were performed by motorized means, now seem to be difficult or even pointless. The apparent difficulty to move causes your perceived physical abilities to diminish. This is a simple way of protecting yourself from any risks your system perceives. In other words, normality (in the form of simple physical movement) is now perceived as dangerous due to the new living conditions, leading to even less somatic mobility - just like increasing age leads to a decrease in perceived abilities, and the consequential avoidance of mobility due to growing fear of injury. The mechanism is the same.

Crucially, the response of your body has changed each time it has to move. Simply walking, even a level road, is often challenging. The message sent by a body that does not move much (experiencing a low fitness level) is to stop and return to inactivity, as soon as possible. It knows so well this inactive state. This increasingly diminishes both physical abilities and the myriad energy-metabolic mechanisms your system uses to sustain life.

More importantly, alienation from exercise causes an even greater loss. During physical movement, the brain produces important neurotransmitters that improve mood and physical and mental health. Most of these neurotransmitters are involved in normal life processes. When their function is disrupted, mental processes such as memory, concentration, and decision-making are impaired.

The further your system alienates from its normal state (i.e., due to unhealthy eating habits, reduced mobility, reduced sleep, increased stress, and other factors), the greater the cognitive disruption gets. Sooner or later, it will begin to send out signals that it is beginning to struggle with its functioning. One such message is what is known as low mood state (also experienced as lack of energy, lethargy, reduced productivity, etc.).

The good news is that normal brain function can be quickly restored through the implementation of helping behaviors. The greater the frequency and number of those helpful behaviors, the quicker your brain will return to its normal functioning.

Frequent physical activity is one of these helping behaviors. Turning physical activity into a daily habit is a key to its successful execution.

The New Habit

Enough about the problem of physical inactivity. Suppose after reading the book in your hands, you decide to add more exercise to your life. How can you do that? What are the steps you need to take?

Most important are steps that lead to the repetition of the behavior in the future, over and over again, without hesitation and exploring what works for you, through what you enjoy.

To understand how this can occur, think about what happens when you face your favorite snack. It may be chocolate, or a flavor you've loved since childhood. It could be your grandmother's favorite pudding or the dessert you want to try every time you walk by the bakery in the neighborhood. What's your reaction? How does your mind manifest its desire to sample that beloved taste again?

This is exactly the reaction you need to have, in order to include regular physical activity in your life. It may not be as strong the first time you perform this activity. Obviously, there is a need for you to keep repeating and persevering.

Here are some simple ideas for your new habit:

1. Make it a priority

What the eyes observe is what the mind perceives. This rule is the foundation of any new habit. See the sports equipment in the car, place it in your bag, or next to the desk. The pair of sneakers next to the front door. Create the shortcut that leads to the gym — not your house — after you leave the office. A date with your girlfriend in the park. The morning workout at the pool with fellow swimmers. All these together, and each of them individually, provide the initial stimulus to start the activity. The more often you repeat it, the greater in significance it becomes.

2. Program it

Exercise is a time commitment, but also a break commitment. A break in your daily calendar. Place it where it's convenient to do it, and where it interferes the least with other things you need to get done. It might be early in the morning, as soon as you wake up. In the afternoon, during a break. In late afternoon or evening, when the main tasks of the day have been already completed.

It is obvious that such a break must be in sync with the other central behaviors you perform: eating, resting, communicating, working, having fun, and sleeping. The more experience you gain in combining your movement activities with these central behaviors, the more in control of your mood you will feel at the end of your day.

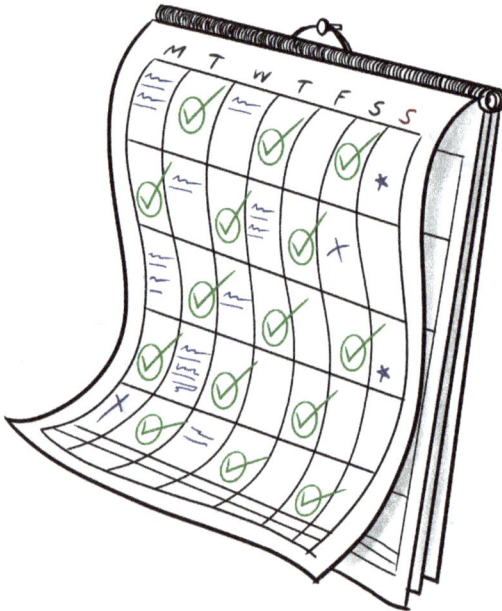

3. Build your routine

Any new activity takes time to establish as a habit. On average, this time is about ten weeks (Lally et al., 2010). The success here is based on sequencing the behavior. In simple terms:

- I organize the equipment, the appointment, or the trip from work to home
- I see the sports clothes, the ball, or the swimsuit
- I have a chat with friends (or individuals that are around and provide an opportunity for a short and genuine conversation)
- I start the activity
- I do it according to my own terms (e.g. according to my physical fitness level)
- I enjoy every moment of it

4. Make it easy

Are the movements you choose easy to perform? Simply put, the more difficult a set of movement activities is for you, the less likely it is for you to repeat it.

For example, consider an activity that you are doing for the first time in a long time: You want to read a book that has been sitting on your bookshelf for long. Play a new game on your phone. Try cooking a recipe you found in a magazine. If you perceive part of the process as difficult, you're less likely to try that activity again — at least for a while, while the memory of that difficulty endures in your mind.

Likewise, the ease of a motor activity is automatically creating a memory trail. Easiness means ability. It translates directly into confidence in how capable one feels on repeating the activity. When your action feels effortless, it gradually becomes repetitive. Repetition provides you with more confidence and competence. Gradually, this leads to improved physical and motor skills, so you can continue to progress your routine.

5. Lower the goal

A difficult goal requires increased motivation. Simply put, a demanding goal requires higher incentives — and more energy — to complete the activity.

That's the exact opposite of what you need to succeed in your new exercise habit! What will give you a fresh start each time you perform a movement sequence, sport, or dance is a low threshold of motivation. A simple and easy task becomes manageable, frequent, and doable.

A simple example: you find that walking for five minutes after your main meals reduces insulin secretion by one third (Buffey et al., 2022), thereby reducing your risk of any blood sugar complications (as overproduction of insulin due to elevated blood sugar is toxic). If you don't walk a lot and want to incorporate this little walking into your schedule, there is no need to start with setting high goals of at least 150 minutes of walking per week (see the WHO guidelines in the How Much Exercise Do You Need section of this book). If you set yourself a high goal (e.g. 30 minutes per day), it means that you will need a high level of motivation to achieve it.

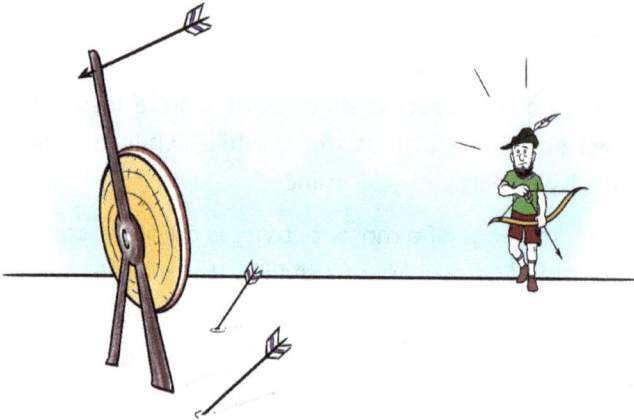

On the other hand, if you decide to take a walk around the block in your neighborhood after your main meal, that walk is easy and without much thought. Instead of sitting in the chair after finishing your meal, you simply put on your shoes and you take a walk around the block. You might run into neighbors you didn't see during the day and hear their news, observe what the weather is like, notice something you haven't seen before. Or you can just walk around without your mind being distracted by bothering thoughts or any of the problems you need to solve.

All of this is helpful. The more often you do this walk, the more you will reinforce this new, easy habit that does not require any encouragement and motivation to take place.

6. Get the Reward You Deserve

Soon your system (the brain and the peripheral, including neuromuscular system) will begin to reward you. No matter when this may happen, fun and pleasure must come first.

What is the activity you can do with ease? And which, as you are performing it, you enjoy every moment? Whether in the company of your loved ones, listening to your favorite music, or out in nature?

Your favorite sport and its characteristics can also entertain you. The speed, the ball, the company, the funny cracks, the ease of doing it, or all of these together can be reasons for fun and enjoyment. The more often you enjoy it, the greater your satisfaction. It is that simple.

7. Choose it

I saved the simplest one for last: the choice. Too often, when you decide what modifications you want to make in your life, you rush into it. You want to change for the better, in the quickest time possible.

In this rush, you decide to do a lot, all at the same time. Improve your diet and fitness, read more, spend less time in front of the TV, pass extra time with the people you love. That's where it gets tricky.

As positive as these changes are, when you begin implementing them, they start competing with each other. Without realizing it, your motivation begins to break down into small pieces. No matter how good you are at doing what you decide to do during each day, something is bound to fall behind. And what gets left behind reminds you that you are not "good enough" to modify properly. You are disappointed. Along with the exhaustion caused by the daily grind, the requirement for increased motivation, and the need for a respite from the constant pressure to achieve transformations, you'll come to stop any effort to improve yourself. It ends up being tougher than you thought it was going to be.

In contrast to the above, choose a behavior, an activity, or one area you want to improve. Focus on the simple, the easy, the everyday, and follow the steps I suggest. The change in your habits will show up sooner or later. Give it the time it needs, forgive yourself if it takes longer than you would like, and show yourself the patience you would advise your friends to show themselves. The result will come, and you will be pleasantly surprised at how easily it can be accomplished!

The Benefits of Frequent Physical Activity

I was really impressed when I first overheard their conversation. I was under the table, there in the café. I had my ears wide open in case I missed any information. It was so impressive that I couldn't wait to go for another walk there with the same group of people, to see if I could catch any more of this fascinating, new information. A young friend of the family I live with, started talking about the benefits of frequent physical activity. My guess is that it's fresh in his mind because of his studies. There's no other reason for the amount of detail he mentioned. The more I listened, the more sense it made. I can feel it, too, every step of the way. So, take note of this:

The myriad positive effects of physical activity are important to experience from an early age, as they contribute to positive psychosocial, emotional, and physical growth and development. They prevent developmental disorders and pathologies, both physical and psycho-cognitive.

At the end of development, the maintenance of fitness through frequent physical activity increases well-being and optimism, through its positive effects on psychosomatic functioning. At the same time, it lowers the risks of metabolic problems (e.g. cholesterol increase), harmful behaviors (e.g. smoking), and negative emotions (e.g. depression). On the other hand, it improves working productivity (e.g. reducing stress) as it supports social relations and maintains positive mood states.

As we age, regular exercise helps to strengthen muscle tissue. At the same time, it maintains physiological functions and quality of life; it is considered a key factor for supporting an active lifestyle and social relationships. Social connectedness is considered the most important factor in maintaining good health and quality of life in senior age groups.

Thus, there is no age group that does not receive significant benefits from regular physical activity. From infancy to later life.

In more detail ...

Muscles, myokines and their importance

Muscle is a tissue made up of cells or fibers that produce the energy and force necessary to meet the body's daily needs for survival and movement. They are mainly responsible for maintaining and changing the position of the body, but also the movement of internal organs. Distinct muscle types perform special functions, depending on their location and type.

Skeletal muscles are among the most dynamic tissues you have. They engage and combine at the voluntary (consciously controlled) order you give them to function. They are over 650 different muscles that are called upon to serve you according to your needs, and make up approximately 40% of your total body weight (Frontera and Ochala, 2015; Noto and Edens, 2018).

In contrast, cardiac and smooth muscles are associated with involuntary (unconscious and unaware) contractions (Frontera and Ochala, 2015; Hafen and Burns, 2018; Noto and Edens, 2018). Smooth muscles are found throughout the body and regulate many of the body's subsystems involved in maintaining survival, such as blood circulation, secretion and transport of vital fluids and hormones, and other essential functions (Hafen and Burns, 2018).

Every time you decide to activate your body's muscles, you set the stage for them to function as a secretory organ to produce hundreds of myokines. Myokines are proteins (peptides) that are synthesized and released by myocytes in muscle tissue each time you move. The more regularly and repetitively you move, the greater the secretion of myokines you induce.

These myokines come into direct and rapid contact with all the organs of your system through the bloodstream, causing significant and profound changes in their structure and function. Organs such as the liver, pancreas, stomach, bones, and brain are transformed when they receive these myokines, improving their function.

There is a large number of myokines released by muscles (e.g. irisin, myostatin, decorin) (Lee and Jun, 2019). One of the most important myokines is interleukin 6 (IL-6), which is released into the blood during physical activity and exercise, and has been shown to have multiple effects on your immune and metabolic system (Ellingsgaard, Hojman, and Pedersen, 2019).

Let's start with IL-6

This protein is really fascinating because it seems to be involved in a double role! Let me tell you about Athena, the Greek goddess. In Greek mythology, she is a goddess with incredible power and energy. She was so powerful, in fact, that she could even overcome the petrifying power of Medusa, who killed with her gaze. I'd like to take a moment to tell you the lovely story of Athena and Medusa, because it really shows how IL-6 works in your body!

In a wonderful turn of events, Athena, with the help of a kind human named Perseus, vanquishes Medusa, a monstrous figure who was impossible to appease. In gratitude, Athena becomes the goddess of wisdom and war. She's the ultimate symbol of good triumphing over evil, of the best in us revolting against the worst. It's that classic battle between reason and passion, spirit and matter, effort and action versus inaction and lethargy. A story as old as time itself.

It's so clear that there's an astounding parallel with interleukin 6. IL-6 is made by your muscles when you are on the move. The more you move your muscles, the more IL-6 is released into your bloodstream. Just after you've finished exercising, it reaches its peak and has its greatest effects for your body and organs. It's so rewarding when you experience the effects of all that hard work! You're really motivating yourself to improve, and you should feel proud of yourself for sticking with it.

It's amazing to think about all the wonderful effects IL-6 instigates as a result of physical activity. I'd like to illustrate this with three examples:

1. It helps to reduce the amount of fat around your abdomen, which is great news for your overall health. Lots of studies have shown that as people get fitter, their bodies store less fat (or fat cells) (Benatti & Pedersen, 2015). To show how IL-6 can help to reduce abdominal fat, researchers in Denmark used a substance that stops IL-6 from working in the body (called tocilizumab) and compared two groups of obese individuals who were taking part in aerobic activities. The great news is that their results confirmed the importance of IL-6 in reducing belly fat. The only group that lost a percentage of adipose tissue from the abdominal area was the experimental group that did not receive the IL-6 inhibitor drug (Christensen, Wedell-Neergaard, Lehrskov et al., 2018).

2. Various epidemiological studies have found that regular physical activity can help to reduce the risk of at least 13 types of cancer (Moore, Lee, Weiderpass, et al, 2016). The good news is that several recent studies have shown that people diagnosed with breast, colorectal, and prostate cancer have increased survival rates when physically active compared to those who are not (Pedersen, 2018). I'm sure you'll be interested to hear about some related research that used the same process of IL-6 inhibition in mice. The results were very encouraging: it seems that IL-6 proteins fight cancer cells while at the same time, they activate specific immune cells (NK) that also target and destroy cancer cells (Pedersen, 2018). Isn't that wonderful? It's so great to see how physical activity can really help to protect you against even such a disease. It helps to boost your quality of life and even your survival rate!

3. Have you ever wondered why it's important to eat slowly? It's because the rate of gastric emptying (the speed at which food leaves the stomach and enters the small intestine after a meal) is the most important regulator of postprandial glucose. This simply means that the slower food transports after each meal, the lower the increase in blood glucose (Woerle, Albrecht, Linke, et al. 2008). I'm happy to inform you that a series of studies with individuals in your species have shown that higher levels of IL-6 slow down the rate of gastric emptying, which helps to keep your blood sugar levels steady after a meal (Lehrskov, Lyngbaek, Soederlund, et al, 2018). The good news is that lower blood glucose levels mean less insulin secretion, which in turn means better health through the reduction of metabolic risks that come with your modern lifestyle. And there's more! The wonderful news is that this effect happens *in addition* to the daily improvements of glucose absorption that occurs as a result of frequent physical activity. It takes place every single day you choose to move sufficiently. With every exercise repetition this protection gets more established, providing further protection to the health of your tissues.

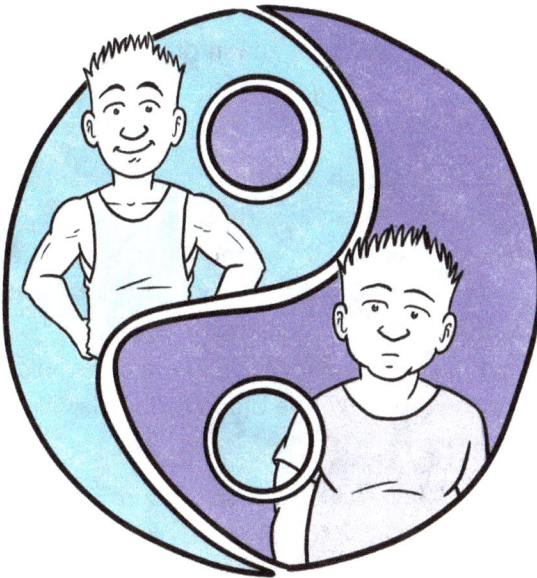

However, your system also produces IL-6 in response to increased inflammation of one (or more) of your bodily functions, even when there's no physical activity involved. In this case, IL-6 is produced by macrophage cells (a type of white blood cell of the immune system that helps to fight off any nasty microorganisms, remove dead cells, and get the immune system going) in response to a disease state and conditions associated with metabolic disorders (such as type two diabetes mellitus), increased levels of inflammation, and adipose tissue deposition, etc. The activation of IL-6 in these instances is trying to reduce further metabolic issues and associated diseases. However, this is when IL-6 increases blood glucose, which can unfortunately lead to a reduction in muscle tissue. In these situations, it's helpful to take a specific type of medication that works to reduce the damaging effects of IL-6-related diseases.

It's like the effect of Medusa, which since the ancient times, has killed every creature that crosses her path. Taking this role, IL-6 identifies with all the destructive effects of a disease-ridden sedentary lifestyle and physical inactivity, as well as the behaviors that do not promote the improvement of your system. So, to sum up, the role and action of IL-6 depends on the environment in which it is secreted and the state of the body.

Several studies have shown that being sedentary while not engaging in enough physical activity in daily life can have a negative effect on your health, no matter the age or gender, and has a damaging influence on your system. Not moving enough can make your belly — or your intra-abdominal ('visceral') fat — larger. This then causes a reaction in the immune system, with macrophages (the type of white blood cells I already mentioned) becoming more active.

Unfortunately, when this condition goes on for weeks, months, or even years without changing, it becomes chronic. This then causes other chain reactions, such as sarcopenia (gradual loss of muscle tissue, strength, and mobility, usually occurring with old age) and anemia (not having enough healthy red blood cells in your blood to carry oxygen to your tissues, a condition that makes you feel tired and weak). And there's more. Insulin resistance and type two diabetes increase also the risk of atherosclerosis (deposition of fat, cholesterol, and other components in the walls of your cardiovascular system). Gradually, brain neurons are equally affected, causing them to degenerate, which can lead to dementia and reduced brain function (Ellingsgaard et al., 2019).

The great news is that you can turn this whole process around, improve your health, and avoid these risks. However, it's very important to remember that reversing this process takes small, frequent, and steady steps, with each of these steps feeding into the new, positive reality that you want to create for yourself.

It is of vital importance to make sure experiences during this process remain pleasant and positive. Any abrupt or threatening practices will damage this course. The wise Ancient Greeks described it so well: «συν Αθηνά και χείρα κίνει» ("God helps them that help themselves"). Or, to put it another way, there is a need to assist yourself by making the changes you aspire to live. You need to tap into the supreme power, the universal energy, or the god you believe in. But above all, you need to be willing and ready to change.

But now let's see if I remember everything mentioned during the lovely chat in the café, and what happens in your system every time you choose to swim in the Magic Lake ...

Physical exercise (and regular physical activity) protects the precious membranes in your body

Human health is linked to the integrity of its membranes at the level of organelles (mitochondria and cell nuclei), cell membranes, internal membranes (between the blood and the brain), and membranes protecting against the external environment (intestinal, respiratory, and skin). Exercise offers significant health benefits by helping to maintain their integrity in the following ways:

- Mitochondria are known as the energy factories of cells, because they are the intracellular organelles that convert the food you eat and the air you breathe into energy, to carry out critical and life-sustaining processes in the body. Two of those procedures are the replication and propagation of DNA, and the synthesis of proteins. Mitochondria produce 90% of the body's energy, so their function is therefore considered vital to human health and daily vitality. During physical activity, there is an increased demand for energy (expressed in the form of ATP), which increases mitochondrial function and maintains the antioxidant function of your system.

In more detail, the mitochondria located within the muscle cells are greatly benefitted by aerobic exercise, improving the structure of their membrane and, consequently, their operation. This improves cardiovascular function and energy transfer, resulting in significant increases of perceived vitality and quality of life (Zhao, Zhang, Zhou, et al, 2020).

- Improving body functions through exercise strengthens the blood-brain barrier, which protects the brain from toxins and immune system cells that can potentially damage it. This provides a unique environment for brain neurons and other brain tissues (i.e. 'white matter') to function well. This barrier plays also an important role in the management and delivery of nutrients to the central nervous system (CNS) (Suresh, Cheng, & Su, 2020).

- Exercise has been shown to preserve the selective permeability of this barrier for substances that need to enter the brain or against those which should be deterred. Research has shown that both strength and endurance physical training can prevent the dysfunction of the blood-brain barrier, even when conditions like inflammatory nerve cell diseases (multiple sclerosis) create significant risks for its potential, by reducing the progression of the disease. In addition, exercise can protect against permeability disorders of this barrier, which are often caused by substance abuse (Małkiewicz, Szarmach, Sabisz, et al., 2019).

- The respiratory system is divided into the upper part (nasal passages, pharynx, and larynx) and the lower part (trachea, bronchi, and lungs). The respiratory tract provides a natural secretory and immunological barrier that keeps out harmful substances such as ozone, pathogenic particles, etc. Regular exercise has many health benefits, including various positive effects on people with chronic respiratory diseases. For example, scientific studies assessing the effectiveness of regular aerobic exercise activities have shown its ability to improve respiratory function, reducing dyspnea in patients with chronic obstructive pulmonary disease (Mohammed, Derom, Van Oosterwijck, et al., 2017) and asthma (Hansen, Pitzner-Fabricius, Toennesen, et al., 2020). Therefore, participation in regular aerobic exercise has been suggested to support pulmonary rehabilitation in chronic respiratory diseases, as it reduces inflammation and improves endothelial protection.

- The skin is the body's main defense shield, and consists of the epidermis and dermis. The epidermis is made up of epithelial cells, responsible for protecting against the harmful effects of the external environment, while the dermis, among other components, contains collagen and elastin. Research shows that regular exercise reduces the risk of damage to the integrity of both layers of the skin by at least 20%, while regular aerobic exercise (45 minutes of moderate-intensity aerobic exercise, three times a week for five months) prevents the thinning of the dermis associated with ageing, keeping it elastic and moisturized (Safdar, Bourgeois, Ogborn, et al, 2011). Apparently, it is not coincidental that regular physical activity is associated with better-looking, younger skin!

Regular exercise keeps you healthy by protecting against significant risks

The invasion of pathogens is a constant threat to your health. Lifestyle, including exercise, has been identified as an effective way to protect against viral infections. Scientific evidence supports the effectiveness of regular physical activity, even against threatening viruses such as COVID-19 (Fernández-Lázaro, González-Bernal, Sánchez-Serrano, et al., 2020). Frequent exercise participation also has antiviral properties, contributing to the significant improvement of physiological and functional parameters, even in patients with viral immunodeficiency (e.g. HIV) or acquired immunodeficiency syndrome (AIDS) (Gomes-Neto, Conceicao, Carvalho, et al., 2013). In summary, regular physical activity helps the prevention of viral infections and the treatment of illnesses, contributing significantly to the protection and preservation of your life.

It is widely accepted that the immune system can suppress certain types of cancer, and immunotherapy is recognized as a promising strategy for cancer treatment. Recent scientific evidence suggests that reduced physical activity is a significant risk factor for various types of cancer. In contrast, regular participation in physical activity is associated with a reduced risk of certain cancers, including colorectal, endometrial, and breast cancer (Leitzmann, Powers, Anderson, et al, 2015). Exercise can therefore play an important role in cancer prevention and therapy, by improving the effectiveness of cancer treatments and their impact on healthy cells (Campbell, Zadravec, Bland, et al., 2020). Frequent exercise participation can also significantly improve physical and cognitive function during what is considered a difficult time for cancer patients.

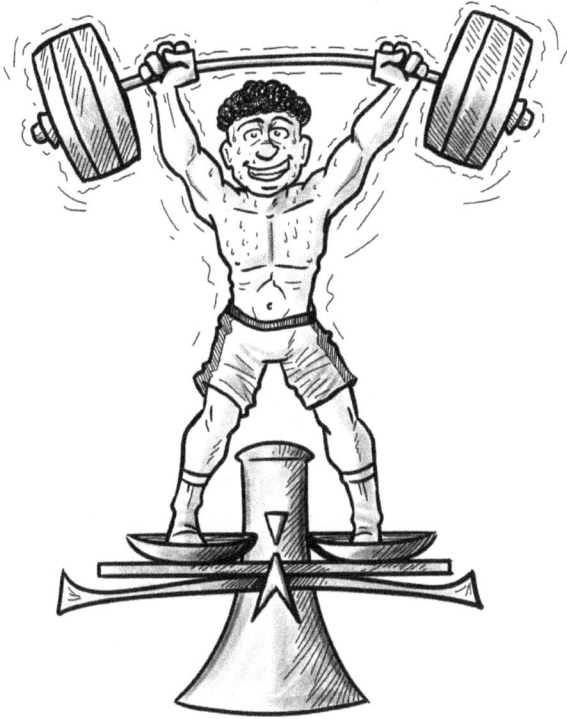

Normal homeostasis is a fundamental requirement for the survival of any organism. It refers to the ability of any organism to maintain a stable internal environment, unaffected by external stimuli (e.g. viruses, external temperature, challenges from external hazards), thus maintaining its equilibrium. However, exposure to the events and challenges of life is not always easy to manage. There are more than a few times when you may feel like your health is being shaken by the circumstances that you are experiencing.

It is therefore important to maintain a positive response to everyday life challenges and their resulting strains on your system. Resistance and resilience to these challenging factors is regulated by many neural, genetic, metabolic, and immunological mechanisms.

Regular exercise significantly improves this homeostatic resilience, helping to maintain good health and quality of life. Exercise and improved cardiorespiratory fitness reduce the risk of a wide range of diseases, including the improvement of functional adaptations in several body tissues (e.g. Deslandes, Moraes, Ferreira et al, 2009).

Some examples on how exercise regulates homeostatic resistance include the following:

- The brain is the primary stress response organ. Stress and stress hormones are a constant challenge to the brain throughout human life. Moderate-intensity exercise improves brain function and helps maintain brain health by inducing a wide range of biological changes in the nervous system. In addition to improved responses against daily challenges, that sustain mental health and positive mood states, beneficial effects of exercise include the improved balance of the autonomic nervous system, better mitochondrial (cell) function, increased neural replication (neurogenesis), improved brain plasticity, and enhanced metabolic fueling — supporting improved angiogenesis and neural health (e.g. Teixeira, Fernandes and Vianna, 2020).

- Regular aerobic exercise and resistance training enhance metabolic health and improve the regulation of the endocrine system. Organs such as the skeletal muscle, liver, brain, and adipose tissue are important metabolic and inter-organ communication components during exercise, helping to improve the homeostasis in the entirety of the human system. Energy demand and consumption induced by regular exercise enhances the use of available energy reserves, including carbohydrates, fat, and glucose, both during and after exercise. This mobilization causes significant changes in many systems, including the endocrine system (Lanfranco and Strasburger, 2016).

- The immune system is designed to respond to any attack

from pathogens that may threaten cellular homeostasis. Changes that occur in the body due to long-term, moderate-intensity exercise are highly beneficial to the immune system, as they increase both the capacity for immune surveillance (against invaders) and immune competence (directly responding to and destroying any pathogens). Hence, regular exercise leads to an improved anti-inflammatory capacity, which is a critical factor in maintaining your overall health — especially against chronic diseases (Petersen and Pedersen, 2005).

-    Your gut microbiota contains many microorganisms that are essential for maintaining homeostasis and normal gut function. The composition of this microbiota is highly variable, and each individual has a unique microbiota profile that plays an important role in their overall health and energy metabolism. The development and stability of the gut ecosystem can be influenced by both endogenous and exogenous factors, including regular exercise and diet.

Regular exercise improves the diversity, composition, and function of the gut environment; moderate aerobic exercise has been shown to increase the number of beneficial microbial species, enriching the diversity of the microbiome and promoting the growth of beneficial bacteria (Clauss, Gérard, Mosca, et al, 2021).

-    Similarly, regular exercise maintains and restores homeostasis at an organic level, by stimulating key physiological adaptations that protect your body cells and tissues from various illnesses. The health benefits of regular physical activity (e.g. 3-5 times per week) include adaptation to repeated metabolic, thermoregulatory, oxidative, and mechanical stressors. For example, it improves energy transfer and use, which increases well-being; it optimizes the ability to thermoregulate during hot summer heat waves or cold winter days by reducing discomfort; and it improves the ability to perform daily movements such as walking, lifting, and carrying goods (e.g. daily shopping, carried out with comfort and reduced risk of injury and musculoskeletal problems). A single session of exercise produces a rapid but transient positive influence in these mechanisms (e.g. at a cellular level), while frequent exercise participation produces significant physiological changes that provide protection against greater challenges or stressors.

This is because exercise induces a multitude of beneficial effects, reducing the progression of diseases through complex interactions between organs such as the muscles, lungs, heart, brain, vascular system, liver, adipose tissue, etc. Consequently, regular exercise is suggested to be the most effective, reliable, and side-effect-free treatment for patients facing surgery. It has several positive effects on the physical condition of patients before surgery, their recovery period, and the length of their hospital stay; improved metabolism, reduced inflammation, and enhanced perfusion (the passage of fluid through the circulatory system or lymphatic system to an organ or a tissue, usually referring to the delivery of blood) of all major organs (Pouwels, Stokmans, Willigendael, et al., 2014).

Your brain

The generation of a variety of neurotrophic (relating to the growth of nervous tissue) factors is thought to be the central mechanism that causes the multiple benefits of exercise on your brain function. Exercise has been shown to be associated with an increase in neurotrophic factors, including brain-derived neurotrophic factor (BDNF), and a reduction in insulin-like growth factor one (IGF-1) and vascular endothelial growth factor (VEGF). All of these promote neuroplasticity and neurogenesis in the hippocampus, the brain area associated primarily with memory (Maass, Duzel, Brigadski et al., 2016).

Brain-derived neurotrophic factor (BDNF) is the most important neurotrophic growth factor, essential for the survival, development, differentiation, and synaptic plasticity of your brain neurons (Taliaz, Stall, Dar, et al., 2009). It is particularly important to highlight that it has been found to be involved in neurogenesis and myelin (myelin is a fatty, insulating substance that wraps around the axons of neurons, protecting them from dysfunctions) repair during adulthood (Khorshid Ahmad, Acosta, Cortes, et al., 2016).

BDNF is widely expressed in your central nervous system, with particularly high concentrations in the hippocampus and cerebral cortex (peripheral region of your brain). Decreased levels of BDNF are found in many neurodegenerative and psychiatric disorders, but even in those cases, systemic exercise causes an increase in this neurotrophic factor, both in the circulation and in the brain, with several beneficial effects occurring for physical and mental health (Dinoff, Herrmann, Swardfager et al., 2018).

Exercise and emotional disorders

Emotional disorders (e.g. depression or severe anxiety) are unfortunately becoming more common in your modern society. There are many reasons for this, with the most important known ones being social alienation, pressuring occupational contexts, sleep deprivation, the use of new technologies and social media, and the reduction of physical activity.

Irrespective of the etiology, mood disorders now affect one in five of your kind worldwide, and are on the rise (Hasin, Sarvet, Meyers, et al., 2018). They are one of the major morbidity issues, often leading to serious illnesses and risks of life. Medications are the most common treatment methods, with psychiatric specialists having the primary role on their type and dosage.

Unfortunately, drugs are not always the answer, as they have many side effects, are not the best treatment for sufferers of mild or moderate emotional disorder symptoms, they often require increasing doses to continue being effective, and are not recommended before the end of development (after 18 years).

It is therefore necessary to have alternative methods that either boost mood or enhance the effect of the medication, gradually reducing the dose needed to improve mental health. Frequent physical activity and exercise is one of the best ways to achieve this result.

A large number of studies have shown that regular physical activity has multiple positive effects on emotional mood, improving mental health responses for 30% to 79% of patients (e.g. Morres, Chatzigeorgiadis, Stathi, et al., 2018) and enhancing the response to psychiatric medication (Rahman, Helgadóttir, Hallgren, et al., 2018). The best evidence for the positive effects of regular physical activity comes from a long-term examination of over 1.2 million adults, who showed significantly improved mood states on physically active days compared to days without aerobic activity or training (Chekroud, Gueorguieva, Zheutlin, et al., 2018). The physical activities that showed the greatest improvement were team sports, cycling, and other aerobic activities, as well as gym activities lasting at least 45 minutes and repeated three to five times per week.

The same results have been seen regarding schizophrenia support, where regular physical activity enhances medication responses, and also provides one of the best solutions against the problem of weight gain that occurs during the treatment of this condition (Dauwan, Begemann, Heringa, et al., 2016).

Physical Activity and Dementia
It is estimated that between the ages of 70 and 74, 3% of your species have cognitive problems. Between the ages of 75 and 89, this figure rises to 22%, and from the age of 90, it reaches 33%. With the increased longevity of your population, it is predicted that cognitive problems will triple by 2050, with ten million new diagnoses of cognitive impairment each year (WHO, 2022).

Despite billions spent on research to find ways to treat

dementia and cognitive decline, regular physical activity remains the only protective mechanism against the biggest disease threat to older people. Several studies, including longitudinal studies and meta-analyses that pool research results together, have shown strong evidence that physically active adults with normal cognitive function are less likely to develop cognitive decline or dementia in comparison to those who are physically inactive. The protection against cognitive decline ranges from moderate (28%) to high (45%), depending on the fitness level and the type of cognitive disease (Alty, Farrow, & Lawler, 2020; Kouloutbani, Venetsanou, Markati, et al., 2021). Therefore, higher levels of physical activity appear to be the best protective behavior against the risk of cognitive decline as the age of your species increases.

Frequent physical activity has various positive effects on reducing cognitive decline, but also reduces the risk of various other behaviors or conditions for your system, such as smoking, weight gain, type two diabetes mellitus, depression, and social isolation. According to several epidemiology studies, adhering to a regular exercise program can have a positive effect on these factors and can contribute to a reduction of the incidence of dementia and Alzheimer's disease by at least 35% (Livingston, Sommerlad, Orgeta et al., 2017).

Protective mechanisms of exercise include significant anti-inflammatory effects and induction of angiogenesis when aerobic activities are performed 3-5 times per week for a duration of 45 minutes or more (Kouloutbani et al., 2021). In addition to aerobic exercise, a variety of physical activities, such as strengthening and balance exercises, tend to reduce depression, and behavioral and mobility problems in people with dementia, who also show improvement in emotional health and sociability.

This is because exercise helps the neurons in the brain to function normally. As previously mentioned, myokine which is the protein released by the muscles when they are activated, which causes a variety of beneficial changes. One of these is an extended neuronal stimulation during motor activity and exercise, that causes various beneficial effects in the brain by changing the activity of brain regions. My understanding is that this causes extensive changes in brain structure and function, including sensitization of membrane receptors, increase in neurotrophic factors (e.g. BDNF) and even improvement in blood vessel structure. These result in an increase in oxygen uptake in the brain (Ganguly & Poo, 2013), as well as an increase in the size of the brain's hippocampus, which significantly improves memory.

More specifically, physical exercise and its effects reduce one of the key mechanisms of dementia initiation, which is related to the deposition of amyloid plaque-induced neurotoxicity, type Ab and tau (Belarbi, Burnouf, Fernandez-Gomez, et al., 2011; Law, Rol, Schultz, et al., 2018).

Exercise and stroke

Stroke is the second leading cause of death in adults worldwide, affecting approximately 15 million humans each year, with 50-75% of all strokes resulting in permanent physical or cognitive disability. A large number of epidemiology studies have shown that patients with cardiovascular disease, diabetes, dyslipidemia, obesity, and reduced physical activity are at increased risk of stroke (Juan, Liu, Willett, et al., 2017).

Frequent physical activity is one of the greatest means of stroke prevention, as its effects include lower body weight, better control of hypertension and glucose tolerance, lower LDL cholesterol levels, and an overall reduction in the risk of cardiovascular disease and diabetes mellitus (Xing Y, Yang SD, Dong, et al., 2018). Clinical studies have shown that people who exercise regularly have a 21% lower risk of ischemic stroke and a 34% lower risk of hemorrhagic stroke (Reimers, Knapp, & Reimers, 2009)!

The benefits of exercise have also been shown during the

recovery from stroke. Regular exercise training after stroke improves walking speed and balance, supports optimal recovery, and promotes an earlier return to independent living, as it contributes to the avoidance of motor and other functional limitations (Tiozzo, Youbi, Dave et al., 2015).

Epigenetics and Physical Activity

We Canis familiaris are the most diverse mammals on the planet. We vary in size, color, behavior, and lifespan as much as any other species (Ruple et al., 2022). But when it comes to our quality of life, we identify with you humans. Our lifestyle, our habits, the environment we live in with its characteristics, the time we spend in nature with its benefits, food types, etc. Our quality of life is largely determined by our healthy years (or the years we live without any manifested health problems). This is called "healthspan".

Of course, our genome (genes) plays a big role in whether we stay healthy or not. The same is true for you. Your genes largely determine who you are.

But in the last 20 years, another important factor seems to have become particularly relevant to the gene-environment-behavior equation. It determines your physical and mental health, and longevity, and is called the epigenetic effect.

The term epigenetics refers to the modulation of the hereditary effect by the expression of specific genes (DNA) from those you have inherited (acting on genes). In simple terms, depending on your habits, choices and lifestyle, different genes will be expressed throughout your life via mechanisms related to methylation (the chemical change in DNA that determines how your cells will reproduce), histones (a key group of proteins for tissue renewal) and microRNA (a mechanism that determines the expression of gene selection in each tissue change that occurs throughout your life).

You may be thinking "what do I care about this process? I care about what happens now". Exactly that. The changes in your cells are happening every day, every single moment, all the time — even this very moment. Right now, as you read this sentence, billions of your cells are being remodeled, reshaping the tissues in all your organs and at every level of your system.

These changes occur as some cells fail or age, and your body replaces them with fresh, new ones that do their job better.

So, on average, each of your 37 trillion cells changes to improve its function at least once every seven years. This means that every seven years you are a new person from head to toe.

Of course, this is a generalization, as your tissues do not change at the same rate and frequency. For example, your skin cells change every few weeks. More specifically, you change 500 million skin cells every day. On the other hand, there are tissues that change at a much slower rate. These include skeletal muscle tissue (essentially responsible for your body's movements), which renews itself every 15 years (Spalding et al, 2005).

The reason I mention this process is simple but very important. The more you follow behaviors that sustain your health, the more your body responds to them positively, further improving your daily wellbeing. Such behaviors relate to healthy diet, physical activity, and even positive emotions or stress reduction.

The result of these behaviors is that your tissues reproduce with the best / improved specifications of your inherited predisposition, improving your organs each time they need to change. Of course, the ability for improving your tissues through the epigenetic process is greater at a young age, but this does not diminish the importance of healthy behaviors and their impact on the epigenetic process throughout life.

Many studies have shown that frequent physical activity has positive effects on your tissues. Put simply, regular physical activity is associated with the expression of better genes every time your cells change, giving you better health. More specifically, in addition to the many positive effects of regular physical activity on your body, frequent exercise activates the expression of genes that support:

- Muscle hypertrophy, fat metabolism, and insulin sensitivity. All of these increase your metabolism and significantly reduce your risk of diabetes mellitus. An example of research with these results is that of Ronn et al. (2013), based on a 24-week regular exercise program

- A reduced risk of chronic disease by promoting the expression of protective genes. An example of such a protective gene expression comes from the evaluation of 25,624 women followed for 13.7 years; those who participated in four hours of regular physical activity per week had significantly lower rates of breast cancer (Thun et al., 1997)

- An epigenetic change that influences the energy metabolism of your offspring. This means that when you participate in a long-term exercise program, apart from the example of positive behavior you set for your loved ones, you increase the protection of future generations against critical metabolic risks (Stanford, et al., 2015). For example, regular physical activity participation followed by both parents before and during pregnancy, is associated with better glucose metabolism, improved neurological functioning, and overall better metabolic health for the fetus and growing infant (Carter, et al., 2012)

- Overall, by supporting the epigenetic process, regular physical activity promotes the expression of genes related to protein synthesis and apoptosis (essential cellular processes for the proper functioning of your body), better mitochondrial function in cells (providing improved energy metabolism and increased oxygen uptake), enhanced function of the heart, liver, and pancreas (key organs for improving your health) and better lipid metabolism, which helps prevent major metabolic diseases (protecting against almost all health risks expressed as a result of modern lifestyle) (Ghafouri-Fard, et al., 2022)

Why You're Avoiding Physical Activity

As your best friend, I'm trying to find the answer to a simple but fundamental issue. With all those good effects exercise contributes to your system, why do you enjoy sitting still or doing nothing? In other words, if constantly avoiding swimming in the Magic Lake and lack of physical activity causes so much suffering, shouldn't it be in your nature to crave every opportunity to move whenever you have the chance?

The answer lies in your thousands of years of evolution. Just as survival made you more able than any other creature on Earth to move for days without stopping, so you could find food and survive for the next day, similar forces urged you to stop. Whenever you had the chance. Whenever circumstances allowed you to stop and rest.

Which are the logical explanations for such a tendency to occur?

First reason:

You tend to concentrate on the simple equation of energy in — energy out. When you didn't have to move to find food, gains in energy conservation and the consequential reduction in energy expenditure was too important to ignore. Therefore, with the obvious gain of energy conservation and survivorship in mind, you chose sitting over other available behaviors (Cheval, Radel, Neva, et al., 2018). Reduced energy expenditure (1.3 fewer calories burned per kilogram of body weight per minute, compared to walking!) may be the main reason you prefer sedentary behaviors to physical activity in the current era.

Second reason:

In the same way you used to spend a large part of your day hunting for food, during most of your evolution and for thousands of years, so did other animals. Hence, it's likely that the more exposed your ancestors were, being outside of their shelters, the more likely they were to fall prey to their predators. The snake, for example, hunts and attacks its prey when it moves unsuspectingly. On the contrary, when you are sitting, you can concentrate better on the stimuli around you, observe what you see, listen to sounds, and smell other creatures around you. Scientific evidence from experiments of your species suggests that everything tends to be better perceived when you are sat, confirming your ability to respond immediately when you are in position to control the stimuli around you (Yue & Quinlan, 2015).

Third reason:

A sitting position reduces the risk of injury. Walking, and especially running, is associated with an increased risk of injury, such as ankle sprains and possible limb fractures, compared to the safety of sitting. In eras when having the time to heal from these injuries was very unlikely, such events would have been fatal. Hence, if there was the option of remaining in a sitting or reclining position, enjoying the safety of others around a bonfire or within the tribe, it stands to reason that there would be an advantage in terms of survival, safety, and social interaction. Thus, mortality risks while living in a dangerous environment probably provided a much stronger selection pressure against physical activity, with related implications for energy balance. However, the ever-needed requirements for food supplies was so great that physical activity was happening during most hours of the day. As a result, this energy balance was always negative, and for thousands of years increased energy storage — contributing to overweight and obesity — was highly unlikely.

These were the living conditions of your ancestors. Surviving is now much easier. However, the problem is that the evolutionary desire to live a sedentary, low physical activity lifestyle remains. Furthermore, your food intake is now completely disconnected from your level of physical activity. You can be inactive without dying of hunger. Your ancestors were not able to do this until very recently, even 150-200 years ago.

It is therefore obvious that your genetic heritage is pushing you towards inactivity, and you seem to succumb to it almost every time you have the opportunity. Inactivity is always pleasant and desirable to you, especially when it is combined with an interesting endeavor such as social connection, storytelling, and your personal interests. The perfect combination for avoiding the Magic Lake and hesitating to experience it!

So, what can you do?

What is the best way to defy the tendency to live an inactive life? Looking at the past — and what kept you physically active — could unlock the solution, allowing you to understand your choices today. You will be able to do so, just like your ancestors. They had no choice but to avoid a sedentary lifestyle; they had to find food to continue to live. They had to move to find their next meal, surviving by helping themselves and each other.

Such impulse is perhaps the solution to inactivity today. No need for any extreme, unbearable, or difficult behaviors, of course. Any compulsion you may create in the current era is much smaller and more manageable than the need to move to survive.

For example, choose to climb one or more staircases instead of taking the lift. If you are using public transport, get off one or more stops before your destination to walk more during the day. Enjoy your coffee with a friend as you are having a walk in a nearby park, instead of sitting in a café. The list is long, and the ways to enhance your daily physical activity, forcing yourself to move, are even longer.

What Prevents and What Enhances Regular Physical Activity?

From what I hear about you, despite that fact that you are aware of the multitude of positive effects derived from regular physical activity, physical activity remains out of reach for a large number of your species. The reasons for this are varied, including the fact that it can be hard to fit exercise into your daily schedule.

I completely understand; with so many pressing commitments, how is it possible to plan a physical activity or a walk, when you are in a hurry to catch up with everything else in the day? The difficulty is great, and the result will always be against you in terms of getting even simple types of physical activity done.

At first glance, this is all true. Your busy schedule doesn't leave much room for regular physical activity. However, if you start to look at your daily habits, you are likely to start to think differently.

Habits are hard to change. This is what the Anglo-Saxons suggest: "You can't teach an old dog new tricks." It obviously means that most of us, regardless of species or background, are reluctant to change old habits or long-held beliefs.

The main reason is that they are comfortable; if they weren't comfortable, they wouldn't become habits. So, by definition, to create a change in our (and your) daily routine, it has to be equally convenient and cost-effective, and should be easy to perform. Finally, this new habit needs to performed frequently, and without having an impact on the rest of the day's activities.

For example, if we look at the amount of time spent watching television, according to the Eurobarometer (2022), the average European watches at least 235 minutes, or just under four hours, of television every day. In Greece, this figure rises to 308 minutes, or more than five hours a day. Even if this figure is not accurate for many, it is an indication of the period you like to spend on relaxing leisure activities in your daily life.

Looking at the scientific literature, the main barriers to regular physical activity in adulthood are related to reduced enjoyment while doing the activity, lack of time and energy, lack of interest, low levels of perceived health, low self-confidence, lack of social support or companionship, poor or old equipment, lack of knowledge related to exercise programs, and poor weather conditions (Dunlap and Barry, 2011).

In comparison, the main reasons for doing various forms of physical activity, relate to enjoyment, social connection, social encouragement, and intrinsic motivation — meaning that the reasons for doing the activity are identified with personal motivations such as fun, better mood, and personal improvement, rather than socially related motivations such as acceptance, admiration, appearance, etc. (Hirvensalo and Lintunen, 2011).

Regardless of the past experiences that determine your next choices, I am hearing that there are critical periods and major life changes that influence your intentions, desires, and behavioral choices. What happens during those?

Critical periods of change
Some of the best-known and most important periods of change in your life as a human being relate to certain ages (e.g. 18, 30, 40, 60), marriage, pregnancy, and the birth of your first child, the end of your studies, a change of job or career, a move to another geographical area, the loss of significant people, and retirement. At many of these critical junctures, the impact is positive. However, whether they affect you positively or negatively depends on your personal reactions and the perceived impact they have on your life. Apparently, research has shown that they can potentially have a significant negative impact on mental health (Moustafa, Crouse, Herzallah, et al, 2020).

In most cases, there are significant benefits to maintaining regular physical activity during these critical periods of change. The first reason relates to its positive effects on physical and mental health, which I have already summarized. A second and equally important reason is the maintenance of a stable routine, which becomes a point of reference in times of significant change. When everything around you is changing rapidly and the old conditions are a thing of the past, a minimum period of absolute control during physical activity provides an important service in maintaining optimism for the future.

Exercise and sport research has shown that after the age of 20, active participation in different sports or regular physical activity declines significantly (up to 50%), especially in team sports. In other words, major life events, professional life, and other significant changes greatly reduce participation in regular forms of physical activity (Lynn, 2010). In Europe, after the age of 50, the percentage of people who regularly participate in these activities *at all* is less than 20% (Eurobarometer, 2022). The problem of reduced physical activity is so significant that the World Health Organization reports that 500 million people in 194 countries are at risk of developing chronic diseases, attributed solely to this reason.

Is it possible to reverse this trend? Is there a hope for you and your peers in the face of modern society's age-related decline in physical activity?

The difference is in the incentives

As far as I know, there is a lot of research that shows that the experience of physical education at school age shapes the way you perceive participation in physical activity. In most cases, the competitive nature and grading style of physical education are not conducive to creating positive experiences that contribute to continued participation in physical activity programs. Similarly, the experiences and knowledge often gained as a student in primary, secondary, and higher education do not match the knowledge needed to continue being physically active for the rest of one's life.

Important areas of knowledge for maintaining good physical and mental health relate to having fun using the body and its capabilities, the importance of self-confidence for body functions and characteristics, and the appreciation of the variety of motor activities needed for supporting good fitness levels throughout life. Similarly, the importance of other central behaviors such as healthy diet, adequate sleep, positive social relationships, etc., can significantly improve quality of life both during developmental years and throughout your lifespan.

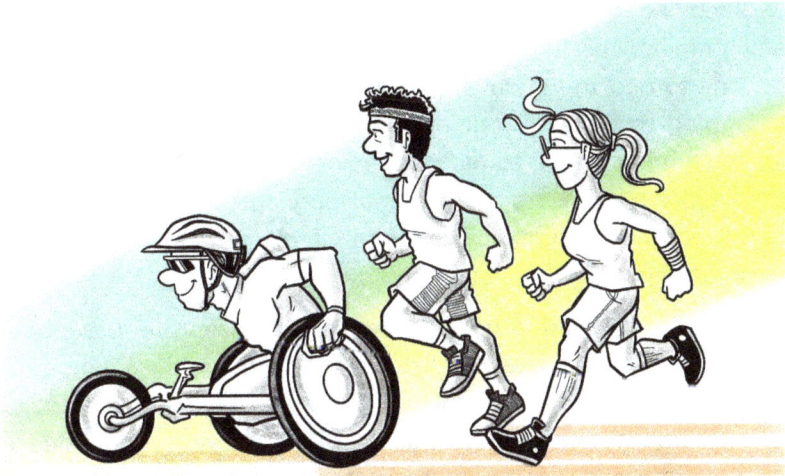

What is motivation?

From the little things I know as a dog, the word motivation comes from the word 'motivus', that denotes the activating processes of psychological motivation. It is a translation of the Greek word 'parakininis' composed of the prefix para-, which means place, next to, before, like, or similar, and the word 'kinisis' ('movement' in English), which refers to action, temporal continuity, and staying in motion. Its ancient Greek root is parakineo / parakino (para + kineo / kino), which means encouragement by words or deeds, the creation of suitable conditions for a particular action, and the existence of a motive for engaging in an action and activity. It is the readiness to act that always modifies the chances of achieving a desired outcome.

Environmental, individual, and interpersonal motivation are important encouraging factors for participating in physical activity. They link different characteristics of human functions and abilities to the performance of a motor task, increasing its frequency and duration.

Speaking of motivation, it is important to start with the environment and its characteristics. For example, if I don't find anyone to accompany me when I go for a walk, there's no way I'm going to feel like running and playing. Without other dogs with a similar desire to play and chase, I get bored. The whole experience becomes a repetition of previous practices. I satisfy my needs and return home. I don't feel any incentive to run, jump, and play.

Hence, speaking from personal experience, social support during a physical exercise can be the key to initiating and maintaining activity throughout the day. The need for social reinforcement is especially important if you have low confidence or certainty around the motor activity you can do. Involving people important to you (e.g. a group of friends or a coach) can enhance your personal expectations of what and how much you can do kinetically. Just being in the same place with your loved ones can provide reassurance and support, reducing any difficulties you may encounter with these activities. Thus, social ties and contacts are important motivators for continuing exercise programs, as they satisfy the need for interpersonal connection and communication. This is the way for any type of physical activity to gain meaning and significance.

In the same way, connecting with important people in your environment while performing your chosen activity can be also enhanced through various tangible acts of support. For example, transport to and from the location of the activity, assistance at the gym, help with everyday tasks such as childcare, simple reminders about the planned activity and, in general, any type of support that helps to make daily participation in physical activity a habit. Any help is welcome if it supports and reinforces your chosen activity.

Similarly, environmental stimuli can be an additional incentive to participate. A new piece of sportswear or accessory often makes the activity not only more attractive, but also more comfortable and safe. Sports clothes and accessories are a reminder and an additional proof — even to you who purchased those in the first place — that this type of physical activity is a personal choice and investment. Even the routine before or after the activity can be combined with added enjoyment and reward. For example, a short break from the daily grind or a bath with your favorite bubbles can be powerful incentives to participate.

Are there any other self-care activities that you find enjoyable during your day? Do you really have any other activities that contribute so much to your self-care like a physical activity of your choice? And are there any other activities that contribute so much during a break from your daily routines? Your chosen physical activity provides clear positive messages on your skills, your physical abilities, and your achievements while relying on your own efforts.

The place where the physical activity takes place can be an additional incentive to participate. Every moment I spend in the park refreshes me. I feel like a different dog. The contact I have while in nature, in a forest, green space, or park, the formations of clouds in the sky, the sun with its beneficial properties, the smells and sounds of nature, are all reasons to exercise outdoors when the weather conditions permit it.

In the same way, when I am in a clean and well-maintained space, I feel so rich and well-treated, like I imagine what being a human would feel like. So, the environment of a gym — safe and stylish facilities, a clean and well-maintained setting, attractive wall decorations, enjoyable music, advanced exercise equipment, nicely designed social and leisure areas, and other types of infrastructure — are all equally important motivators for you humans to start and continue exercising. All these conditions, combined with the instructors' guidance and well-designed exercise classes, enhance even more the motives to participate in physical exercise programs.

The information I have gathered informs me that because of the time constraints you have in your daily living, the proximity of the place you perform your physical activity is another important motivating factor. Related scientific literature has shown that if the area you perform your physical activity is near the place you live (e.g. up to three km away), you are more likely to participate in this form of exercise (Reimers, A. K., Wagner, Alvanides, et al., 2014).

However, before you decide to buy a treadmill or other exercise equipment for your home, it is advisable to try it out and make sure you enjoy this particular form of exercise. Although the home environment seems to be the ideal place for you to increase your exercise participation (due to time saving and proximity), this type of exercise equipment often ends up being used as a clothes hanger or household furniture. This is because your system tends to identify the home environment as a dedicated space for rest and relaxation, which is not always conducive to the choice of exercise activity you want to perform.

Music calms and relaxes us dogs (Lindig, McGreevy, & Crean, 2020). It appears that music of your choice is similarly important during exercise, and is a particularly effective motivator for successful performance during many types of exercise. It is associated with a variety of positive physical, psychological, and psychophysiological effects, as it provides rhythm, increases psycho-emotional tension, enhances your physical responses (e.g. adrenaline release), and improves your mood and well-being (Ekkekakis, Hartman and Ladwig, 2020). And through distraction mechanisms, it also improves your physical performance in activities that require strength, endurance, and speed (Terry, Karageorghis, Curran et al, 2020).

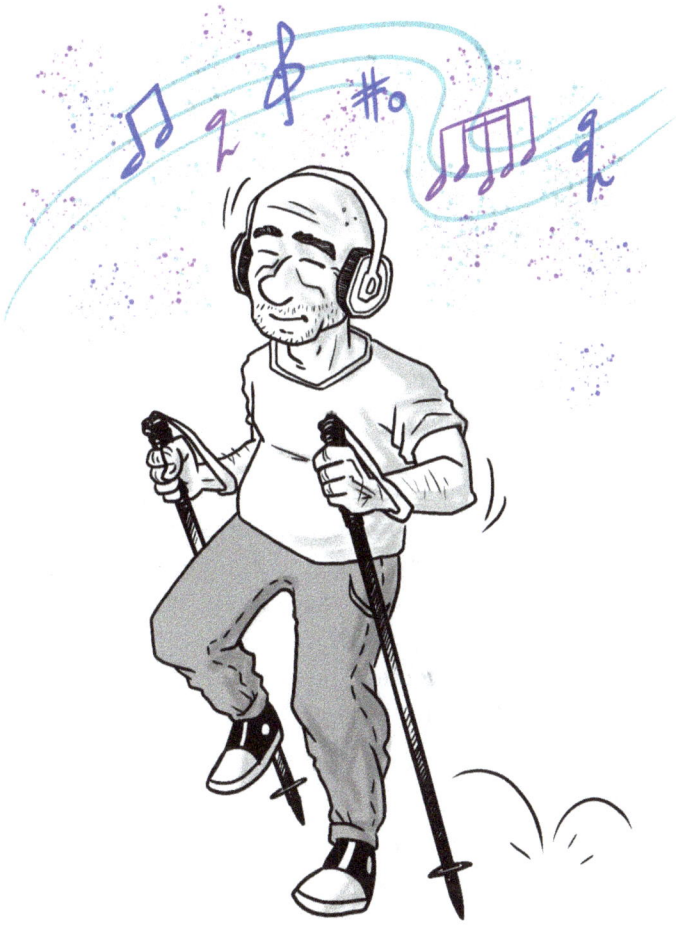

What enhances motivation for physical activity?

The connection with the body and its abilities

I'm sure of myself. I can run, play, catch my ball, jump high, chase cats. But if there is a bigger, louder, or rowdier dog in the park, I hang back until he leaves. I don't go looking for trouble; I know those guys. After all, I'm in the park to have a good time, not to get in a fight.

Something similar happens to you and the rest of your kind. Every attempt you make at physical movement requires the use of your body and its parts, your physical self. This requires a connection to your available — actual or perceived — physical capacities.

Here lies the complexity of the unique connection with your body and the abilities you perceive you have at any given moment: previous experiences influence this connection, as each person forms a personal appreciation of the required movement and its parts. Whenever you are asked to perform a series of movements, to influence your environment by performing every day necessary activities, or to perform actions that are part of a particular series of exercise activities, you weigh up the demands of the movement based on previous experiences. In the blink of an eye, you are considering the length of time you have not performed a similar movement, your current abilities, how your body feels, the environment, any bystanders, how others who have performed this movement have executed it, etc. It is all part of the theory of self-efficacy.

Self-efficacy

In 1977, to explain human behavior and its motivators, Bandura made a series of theoretical proposals that strengthened behaviorism with cognitive elements, accepting the importance of personal thoughts in human decisions. To explain the perceived and personal expression of the ability to act and influence one's environment, Bandura (1977; 2018) formulated the theory of self-efficacy, which refers to each individual's belief in their ability to perform necessary behaviors to achieve certain outcomes (Bandura, 1977, 1986, 1997).

Self-efficacy reflects confidence in the ability to control personal motivation, behavior, and the social environment. These continuous self-evaluations influence all kinds of experiences and behaviors, including the goals you set, the energy you expend to achieve those, and the likelihood of achieving certain levels of performance.

For example, perceived ability is directly influenced by the way other people with the same characteristics as yourself tend to behave, and by the popularity these individuals seem to have. Your likelihood of adopting their behavior depends on your personal characteristics, the elements of the environment in which you find yourself, and your previous behavior-related experiences.

Consequently, according to self-efficacy theory, whether you will engage in a particular behavior depends on what other popular people in your immediate or wider environment are doing, your previous experiences of the behavior (successful or not), the influence of your environment through the direct or indirect messages it provides, and any physical experiences and emotions produced when you engage in that behavior. The more positive these messages are, (e.g. the more they provide conditions for success, creating relevant expectations of achievement), the more likely you are to perform the behavior. The applications of self-efficacy theory to the exercise behavior are obvious:

- Your previous successful experiences prepare you for the next movement stages, and relates goals

- It is crucial that important people in your social environment reinforce physical activity through their behavior and beliefs

- It is essential that your readiness for a new (e.g. longer, more challenging) physical effort is not affected by previous negative emotional and somatic experiences

- Verbal reinforcement, appropriate instructions, and the camaraderie of others (i.e. active exercisers) are likely to inspire and persuade you to perform increasingly difficult motor activities

According to researchers, you have two types of self-efficacy: the first type relates to the belief that you can successfully perform a motor activity (e.g. of a certain type, duration, intensity, and difficulty). This is obviously important for the expectation of success, and the progression of goals and difficulty levels associated with your motor activity.

However, the second type is equally important as it relates to your ability to create the conditions for performing the motor activity in your daily living. When you consider what you need to improve based on your fitness level, doing a simple exercise program once a month or once a week, regardless of its difficulty levels, is not going to improve your skills enough to be a reason to continue (e.g. realizing an improved quality of life). Rather, your ability to cope with the challenges of everyday living, scheduling physical activity as frequently as required (i.e. three times a week), is an important prerequisite for success in achieving these goals. In the same way athletes need to improve under all possible circumstances to achieve desired performance, there is a need to cope with the ever-changing elements of your daily living that could interfere with your physical activity plans to be able to execute those effectively.

It's important to remember that it's not easy to perform and regularly repeat physical exercise programs. That is because exercise is not a simple automated behavior that starts and ends in a few minutes, such as brushing your teeth.

To perform physical activity regularly, you need to organize and execute many different skills. On a first level, there is a need to fight the resistance you may feel by competing against daily habits that may be antagonistic to regular exercise plans (e.g. watching TV in the comfort of the sofa at home, or a friendly get-together). Following that, you need to combine behaviors aiming towards the goal of becoming more physically active; join a group that does the exercise you enjoy, regularly pay an amount of money (i.e. a monthly subscription to a gym), have special equipment to perform the activity, and be able to successfully complete a challenging program for your fitness levels. Similarly, until the expected physical and mental improvements occur, you may feel intimidated by some elements of the exercise environment (i.e. other individuals being more popular due to their abilities and skills), and the immediate effects of exercise on your system (e.g. muscle soreness and fatigue).

Some important questions you need to answer to increase your self-efficacy levels are;

- Can you dedicate 30 minutes in your daily schedule to exercise?

- What time of the day is best for doing that, based on your schedule? (Think of a time slot that is less likely to clash with other important activities in your day)

- What are the activities that may put at risk, sabotage, or cancel your planned physical activity regime?

- Are there times in the day that you spend commuting, queuing, or pausing which could be used for short bouts of physical activity?

- Which are the most frequent reasons for cancelling the exercise or other activities you enjoy? For example, caring for children or loved ones, holidays, or travelling, can be significant reasons for cancelling or inhibiting physical activity. Is there anything you can do to change the way you do those?

- Is there a meeting during the day that could be combined with a stroll? A business or social meeting held in a park could be transformed into a leisurely walk, creating better physical and mental states for all stakeholders.

- Finally, family moments and gatherings can be made more enjoyable by combining a walk with movement games, or by using objects in the environment for organizing games or quizzes that inspire young and older alike (for examples of such games, see: http://growingfamily.co.uk/exploring-nature/kids-nature-games/)

The importance of self-determination
My daily walks are very different when I'm on a lead. I can't enjoy my freedom of movement, smell where I want, chase the birds, and play with the other dogs. I don't have the same enjoyment of the smells and intense stimuli of the outside world when I'm leashed, restricting every moment.

Something similar happens to you every time your behavior is restricted. It has to do with the extent which important people in your environment determine what you do, and is elucidated by self-determination theory. Let me explain it from the beginning so you can understand it.

Central to self-determination theory is the distinction between self-determined (autonomous) or hetero-determined (environmentally controlled) motivation to participate in physical activity. For example, if physical activity is done to gain the approval or liking of important people around you, the motivation to participate is extremely hetero-determined (hetero-determined simply means that one's actions getting regulated by significant individuals around them (i.e. partner, colleague, medical doctor) and your participation in such activity is not expected to last. It is also called 'amotivation' as a behavior state, meaning the incentives to participate in the activity are quite restricted, resulting in abandoning the activity before long.

At the next slightly higher level of motivation, physical activity takes place when you feel guilty if not performing it. The guilt associated with this motivation exists because many of the positive health effects of physical activity are already known, but you have not yet discovered the elements you can enjoy in the exercise activity (or the parts of yourself that can be expressed through this behavior).

At a next level of motivation, the positive things you experience through physical activity (e.g. the improvement in endurance and strength, reduced stress levels) create the least hetero-determined or environmentally controlled form of motivation. Nevertheless, this form of incentive remains an external motivator, as it does not derive from you but from the activity and the effects it provides to your system.

On the flipside of extrinsic motivation, intrinsic incentives are the most genuine form of motivation you can feel. They refer to all personal reasons you may have for participating in physical activity. They reflect your positive emotions (enjoyment, joy, personal satisfaction, sense of achievement), but also the satisfaction of the genuine and spontaneous social contact you experience during the activity. Such emotions generate the self-determined form of motivation, that is also expressed as a feeling of unique connection with the motor activity you may experience (e.g. absorbing environmental stimuli), and the perceived cognitive and emotional rejuvenation during and after your favorite motor activity.

Many studies have shown that an element of the environment is directly related to these positive feelings: the greater the perceived and actual autonomy offered in the physical activity environment, the easier it is to maintain an increased participation in physical activities. Simply put, the greater the sense of freedom of choice regarding the type, duration, intensity, and frequency each time you participate in a physical activity, the more positive your experience of exercise will be (Hagger & Chatzisarantis, 2008).

Autonomy is also critical for the improvement in ability and skill you experience during the activity. For example, the higher the choice and freedom you have, the greater the sense of improvement in motor and physical skills you feel.

Finally, autonomy, along with social connectedness and competence, are your basic human needs. When these are satisfied or enhanced by the environment of motor activity, the greater the increase in intrinsic motivation you experience. Combined with the positive emotions mentioned above, autonomy creates one of the most successful conditions for increased motivation and continued active participation in exercise programs of all kinds.

What are the characteristics of an environment that satisfies these three basic human needs?

An autonomy-enhancing environment values the individual and their freedom of choice. It emphasizes experimentation, decision making, and personal responsibility. It reinforces the expression of authentic behavior, as well as self-improvement, to continue participation without the need for coercion or the implementation of environmental conditions.

In contrast, the environment that denies autonomy is associated with threats, deadlines, goal setting, control, and constant evaluation of behavior. In such a controlling environment, assessments often take the form of comparisons, having as a reference the performance of others and emphasizing winning above and beyond any other experience. Does this ring a bell? If so, how much time did you spend participating in such an environment, and what do you remember about it?

How does an environment that enhances perceived competence look like? It must include rewards for the pleasure and enjoyment of each activity, especially when these are linked to new successes in learning important activities. This creates a sense of achievement and a need for further development. No matter how many hours you spend practicing, they do not diminish the effort you put in: each new experience is exciting and increases your sense of achievement. If the activity does not provide you with new learning challenges and recognition of your improvement, the environment will not increase your perceived ability. This leads to a reduction or avoidance of further effort.

Finally, social contact is about human nature and fulfilment. It relates to the need for care and love that is inherent in human life. The sharing of thoughts, interests, emotions, and behaviors is a basic requirement for human survival (Gilbert, 2015). Likewise, an environment that satisfies this human tendency provides more stimulation and attracts interest. The absence of discrimination, equal opportunities to participate, mutual support, the continuous development of relationships, and the positive experiences generated by social contact all enhance self-esteem and strengthen coexistence. This is the environment that promotes social contact, and these are some simple ways to increase motor activity and satisfy your need for real social interaction.

Some questions you can answer to find out if your environment is helping to motivate your favorite activity are:

- Are you doing the physical activity because you want to improve elements of your appearance? If so, it is important to combine these appearance motivators with important internal motives related to positive emotions (e.g. enjoyment and satisfaction from participating in the activity) if you intend to continue

- Intense military-style motor activities (e.g. Cross Fit) based on coercion and military orders do not offer opportunities for personal choice, and gradually reduce the motivation to engage in physical activity. Apart from not engaging in the activity for long due to reduced intrinsic motives, there is also a high risk of injury from intense, uncontrolled, and non-individualized exercises

- Do you have a choice about the way you perform your physical activity type(s), promoting self-expression? Does the way you perform your chosen activity offer you alternatives and opportunities for personal choice? If so, you are on the right track

- Do you feel that you are improving through the activity (or activities) you are doing? In which areas? When do you feel this improvement? Is there anything you can do to increase this feeling?

- Do you have opportunities for social interaction and meaningful human contact during your chosen activity? If not, how can you increase these opportunities?

- Do you have the time and inclination to observe the environment and what it offers when you do a physical activity? If not, plan some walks in nature and give yourself time to observe

- Finally, if the environment you find yourself in does not support your basic needs for autonomy, competence, and social contact, it is never too late to search and choose an activity that can satisfy these needs

Here are a few helpful questions that I ask every time I lie down on my favorite spot, listening to the conversations of those who know. They relate to everyday questions you may have about the Magic Lake, and the ways to approach its waters, enter, or swim in its magic environment.

10 + 1 Questions and Answers

1. I'm bored of anything that has to do with physical activity. Do you have any suggestions?

Past experiences often determine your choices. The phenomenon of refusing even the idea of a short walk or more physical activity than the amount you do every day is well known. I'll start with the simple suggestions: not every exercise activity feels the same each day or in different parts of the day. The way you perceive the effort of an activity depends on your level of tiredness or fatigue, the activities you've done before, the way you've eaten and slept recently, the physical and social setting, etc.

For these reasons, better to start moving by doing simple and short activities: walking around the block is enough to get you started. Do this walk when you have time and are not pressured by other commitments. Take your time and notice how your body feels. There is no need to overdo it at the beginning. No need to hurry, or to add time and effort to this simple walk. Allow time to feel the improvements that come by repeating this walk. Choose different routes, visit the park nearby, observe what happens around you. Ask someone close to accompany you, doing the walk together. Have fun.

2. How do I know I'm getting enough exercise to get all the benefits mentioned in the previous pages?

The most important thing about any physical activity is the quality of your experience, for the simple reason that if you don't enjoy it, you won't do it again. So instead of worrying about the physical, cognitive, and psychological improvements that come from exercise, focus on having fun as you experience being physically active.

Put simply, the better the experience you have, the more often you will do it. With increased frequency comes a greater variety of performed physical activities and more positive effects on your system. All of these create improvements to your physical and mental health.

3. What should I do if my body hurts after a walk or when I start a new exercise program?

To answer this question I need to explain some basic principles of coaching. Whenever you perform a motor activity and try to quantify this experience, you will use numerical quantities that describe its duration (e.g. eight minutes), its frequency (e.g. I did this distance four times last week) and its intensity (the difficulty of this activity, e.g. uphill for three minutes). Progressing in each of these metrics relates to your fitness levels. Adding duration, frequency, and intensity to physical activities needs to be gradual, to avoid fatigue and the risk of injury.

I suggest you progress each type of exercise program first in duration (e.g. from eight minutes to ten minutes), then in frequency (e.g. from four to five times a week) and finally in terms of intensity (e.g. uphill for five minutes instead of three). I will now continue this short lesson by explaining the three basic principles of coaching:

A. The **overload** principle, which means that to improve your physical abilities, you need to do an activity that is harder than what your body is used to doing. Avoiding this won't develop any physical ability (e.g. strength, endurance, speed) and your physical capabilities will simply remain at a basic or moderate level.

B. The principle of **progressivity**, explained in terms of the need to develop your physical abilities gradually, i.e. through motor activities that become gradually more difficult and in a sequence that ensures this advancement (i.e. duration, frequency, and intensity), in each type of activity you choose (e.g. walking, swimming).

C. The principle of **specialization**, which simply means that if you perform an activity on firm ground (e.g. walking), the improvement in your physical abilities will be related to moving on a solid environment (as opposed to an icy or fluid one). In other words, you cannot expect to improve your skills in a different environment than the one you are training in (e.g. swimming in open water or in a swimming pool).

The reason behind explaining these principles is to make you aware that it is normal to feel a slight tightness in the muscles after an exercise program that lasts longer than usual, or after a period of not engaging in a particular type of exercise. This is like engaging in physical activity after a long period of inactivity or when doing something more advanced for the first time.

Hence, it is important to know that if you end up with some sort of muscle soreness after an exercise program, it means you've overdone it. The best way to eliminate muscle soreness is to avoid inactivity. Provided that no muscle injury has occurred (an injury is quite unlikely if you have been sensible), performing short, low-intensity movements (for example, light and slow walking for sore leg muscles) will help eradicate any sore muscle symptoms.

To sum up, when your body hurts after an exercise program it is probably due to sore muscles. I am sure you will be able to avoid muscle soreness by giving additional time to improve your physical abilities and using the basic coaching principles outlined above, So, yes to your progress, but make sure it is always gradual.

4. How do I know I am ready to start moving more?

As physical activity is a basic human behavior and essential for sustaining good physical and mental health, it is safe to choose and be physically active every day. However, if for some reason you have not been physically active for long, it is advisable to get your GP or family doctor to certify your readiness to exercise.

Equally, if you have a clinical illness, it is necessary to follow your doctor's opinion on your readiness to start a new type of physical activity. In such a case, it is important to follow the principles of progression, mentioned above.

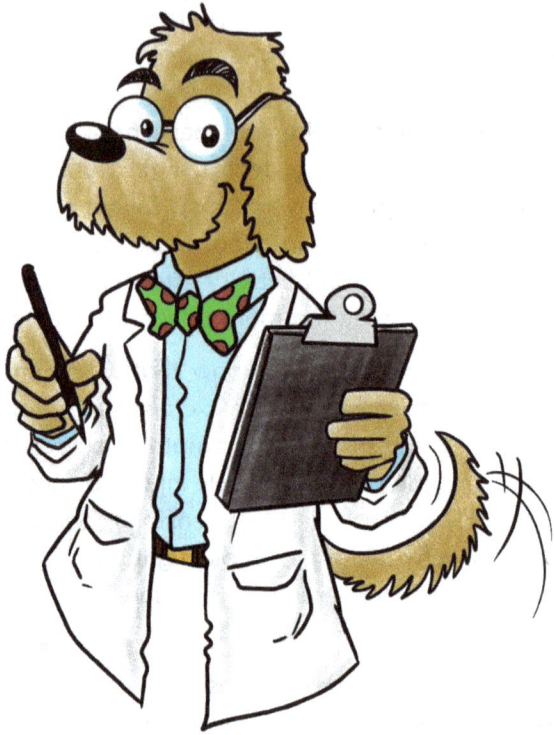

5. Can I trust personal trainers?

In order for an exercise specialist to be able to give you the right scientifically sound advice, it is important that he or she is properly trained and has studied at the highest level.

Scientifically sound exercise advice comes from properly trained experts. Graduates of higher education institutions that specialise in the subject (e.g. a combination of Physical Education and Sport & Exercise Science degrees) are best suited to create a personalized physical activity program based on your needs.

Unfortunately, many of the exercise-related education / training programs preparing their graduates for specific exercise types (e.g. yoga, group aerobic dance programs, etc.) are purposed around the needs of the average healthy exerciser, and do not provide the required knowledge to specialize / individualize exercise programs.

Therefore, before you trust a personal trainer, check their suggestions. Just because they look fit does not mean they have the knowledge to train you safely. Check their expertise and knowledge.

6. When should I expect my body to change through an exercise program?

Improving appearance is often one of the main motivators for engaging in a more physically active life. Yet, for reasons explained thus far, it is not always the best type of motivation for long-term engagement in physical activity.

At an initial level, it can be an important incentive for participating in exercise programs, and could become a reason to continue exercising. Especially if the changes observed are the desired ones.

The problem is that people often have very high expectations related to improving their appearance via being physically active, forgetting that without investing the effort, regularity, and enjoyment, such change is almost impossible to take place.

Creating physical and energy adjustments that can potentially change appearance (e.g. causing weight loss), necessitate engaging in frequent exercise sessions and intensifying previous levels of energy consumption. Such change requires adjusting other daily behaviors like eating, sleeping, working, etc., to accommodate required resources and fitting everything in new daily routine.

Another aspect to consider in such a pursuit is the implementation of different types of exercise programs that can improve and accelerate improvements in physical appearance. Combining an aerobic exercise program (e.g. walking, swimming, aerobics, dancing) with muscle strengthening (e.g. Pilates, fitness bands, body weight resistance) can provide different stimuli, creating better control over one's appearance and enhanced commitment to increased physical activity participation.

Therefore, a successful recipe for improved appearance via exercise participation requires a mixture of regularity, duration, enjoyment, and a variety of movement activities.

7. Should I count the calories I burn through physical activity?

There is a misconception that any calories burnt kinetically correspond to the food types one eats and the calories they contain. Risking oversimplification, this is misleading and inaccurate for two simple reasons:

A. Calories contained in food are used to provide energy to our organs, to keep us alive, to aid digestive processes, to provide energy for motor movements, and to sustain us during fasting periods (Osilla, Safadi & Sharma, 2022). If we eat more energy than our body uses, any excess calories are stored for future use.

B. When we exercise, our body uses some of the energy it needs from the food we have eaten recently (e.g. in the last 24 hours). But after about ten minutes of exercise, we begin to use up the stored energy (e.g. adipose tissue, or fat cells) that remains in our system for that purpose. The longer we exercise (e.g. walking or running), the more we use up this stored energy.

In other words, calories are energy and, of course, when they are ingested, they are not used directly and in their entirety. Hence, there is no need to count the calories one burns through physical activity to make sure they are enough. The reason for this is simply because the idea of burning X number of calories by doing Y number of minutes / hours of a particular type of physical activity, equalizing calories received during a meal, is wrong.

So the most important thing in one's diet is the quality of the calories one receives, as those are the ones giving energy, valuable nutrients, and improved well-being. It is also worth mentioning the value of exercise in appetite control: frequent physical activity makes it increasingly difficult to overeat unhealthy food types that cause metabolic diseases and related health conditions. The reason behind that is the brain and its ability to recognize what is best for our system. Brain centers (e.g. the hypothalamus), perceive that one does not need to store fat, reducing in this way the appetite to consume food types causing an increase of body fat (Blundell, Gibbons, Caudwell, et al., 2015).

8. I have started to move more but I am not losing weight. On the contrary, the scale shows that I have gained weight!

Another misconception is that if the scale shows a lower body weight, one has lost fat. When one steps on the scale, the number they see reflects the weight of every existing tissue type (i.e. bone, muscle, body fluids, fat, etc.) one has.

When one starts undertaking more physical activity, their system creates new muscle tissue from the available amino acids and proteins. That's why it's important to start gradually, so that one's body has time to build up this new muscle tissue, helping to perform a variety of required activities while reducing any risk of injury. This will protect you from any inflammation that may be caused by the sudden realization of new activities and their immediate demands.

In comparison to the fat tissue that one starts to lose as a result of the performed motor activities, this newly created muscle tissue has a higher relative density due to its composition (e.g. various important fluids it contains) and its energy potential. This is because fat is made up of adipose tissue, i.e. it is not hydrated tissue, and beyond a certain percentage necessary to sustain life, it does not promote health.

Therefore, the number on the scale is not an accurate indicator of the positive changes occurring in one's body composition because of physical activity. Measuring adipose tissue and assessing one's body composition is a far more accurate indicator of the changes taking place in one's body as a result of frequent physical activity participation.

9. Sports equipment and sports brands are very expensive. Do I need to buy such expensive sporting gear?

It is true that sports equipment can be quite expensive and is indeed an important expense in the quest for a more active lifestyle. However, beyond the rules of the market, driving up and down the price of products through supply and demand, the value of sports equipment contains other qualities that are important to emphasize, to facilitate one's decision whether to buy a related apparatus.

The products of a well-established sports equipment label or brand are based on years of research and development into new materials, design, technology to protect you as a user, and focusing on your needs. For example, sports equipment designed for inexperienced users has little in common with apparatus designed for experienced exercisers. This obvious difference highlights the importance of sports equipment in preventing injuries and other risks during any sporting activity.

Consequently, a simple answer to the above question is that the purchase of specialized sports equipment is indeed important, and recommended for reducing injuries that may occur during your favorite activity. Simple market research will help you to sort out the price levels of the necessary equipment for your chosen physical activity or sport, so you can decide accordingly based on your needs and budget.

10. Should I try to reach 10,000 steps every time I walk?

Although the daily target of 10,000 steps per day may be a good objective for improving aerobic capacity — along with other fitness skills — it is important to clarify where this number comes from and whether it corresponds to the recommended daily rates of physical activity.

As a matter of historical context, it is worth noting that the importance of physical activity in the fight against lifestyle-related metabolic diseases began to be acknowledged when Japan was preparing to host the 1964 Tokyo Olympics. For all reasons previously explained, the simplest form of exercise is walking. As the average Japanese person was engaging in about 5,000 steps a day at the time, a pedometer company decided to double this figure to give the largest proportion of adults in the country a new objective. This new figure made it easy to promote step counters, and their sales to the general population of Japan soared significantly.

The term *Manpo-kei*, which means 10,000 steps in Japanese, became a catchphrase for dedicated Japanese walkers, and was the minimum they needed to walk to achieve the expected health benefits. Gradually, the 10,000-step goal caught on around the world, and most health experts now recommend it as a key fitness goal for a structured physical activity program.

Despite the popularity — and simplicity — of this step objective for the general public, there are significant problems with its implementation. Firstly, it does not take into account one's initial walking ability and fitness level to set relevant and personalized targets. As a result, there is a risk that one will not be able to achieve this number of steps in a reasonable amount of time and may become frustrated, giving up any effort to engage in physical activity.

Also, assuming that one achieves this number of steps on most days of the week, lacking further fitness goals may lead to decreased motivation and eventually abandonment of the exercise habit (who can continue to perform an activity that does not provide opportunities for further improvement?).

Therefore, the answer to the 10,000 steps question is that one needs to always consider not only their initial level of physical ability, but also their personal preferences to satisfy the personal needs for autonomy, perceived competence, and social contact (see the section on self-determination and its importance for motivation). Also, after the initial assessment and expert approval for initiating an exercise program, selecting the duration, frequency, and intensity of activity should be part of one's personal choice, rather than the experts' appraisal that may limit personal development and motor choices.

Bonus question: my doctor told me to walk often because of a health problem I had. But I'm getting more and more bored of the same old exercise program ...

The previous question and its answer explain how one can increase levels of daily physical activity, regardless of the reasons they have started exercising. It is important to stress that there is often a lack of motivation to continue with these programs. This is because one is often following these guidelines as medical rehabilitation (e.g. heart disease or related surgery). As a result, one is often pursuing other-referenced incentives to participate in these activities, and this could result in the gradual abandonment of the activity since the exercise program does not seem to fulfill personally meaningful motives.

The solution to this lack of motivation is to try to find activities that are more enjoyable (e.g. because of past experiences, it could be that cycling, dancing, or swimming are your favorite activities). It is precisely for this reason that one will likely be able to perform those with greater frequency and for a longer, reaping the positive effects of physical activity.

On the other hand, the freedom to explore one's personal limits in terms of the duration, frequency, and intensity of a favorite activity can bring significant benefits. For example, ten minutes of a self-selected walking activity (e.g. in terms of the route, time, intensity, and breaks) can gradually lead to longer and more variable periods of exercise.

A walking activity can be easily developed into a regular exercise program with a combination of walking and slow running. This can lead to 30 minutes or even an hour of running. After that, where one may choose to develop their personal skills and fitness level is entirely up to personal goals and choices.

Whatever one's reasons for starting to increase their physical activity and exercise participation, it is important to explore personal preferences before they lose motivation risking giving up their newly created physical activity behavior.

A Few Words at the End

That's it, I've told you everything I see in you. What I know that saddens and angers me every time I observe it. The truth is that your nature is complex and multi-dimensional. This, of course, is what makes your daily choices and priorities difficult to determine in advance, without having the necessary self-control.

It's also what makes swimming in the Magic Lake more difficult for you than it needs to be. I hope that through my thoughts I have made clear to you the reasons why it is useful to get wet or to swim in the magical waters of the lake, with the highest frequency you can achieve. I have also mentioned the ways you can make it happen. And, of course, the motivation you need to keep experiencing its miraculous waters.

The daily wellness you may have in mind is probably far from what I think about you, or what science suggests for improving your health. And, of course, it is better for you to appreciate your own needs as they have been shaped by your experiences. Therefore, use the information I've included in this book in the way that makes sense to you.

I hope that you will listen more and more to your body, mind, spirit, and system needs. Alongside this, pay attention to your characteristics and strengths. They make you special. Nurture them as you deserve and claim the best form you can obtain. Swim in the Magic Lake and enjoy every moment.

Bibliography

Alty, J., Farrow, M., & Lawler, K. (2020). Exercise and dementia prevention. *Practical Neurology, 20*(3), 234-240. https://doi.org/10.1136/practneurol-2019-002335 .

Belarbi K, Burnouf S, Fernandez-Gomez FJ, Laurent C, Lestavel S, Figeac M, et al. (2011). Beneficial effects of exercise in a transgenic mouse model of Alzheimer's disease-like tau pathology. *Neurobiology Disorders. 43*(2):486-94 https://doi.org/10.1016/j.nbd.2011.04.022

Benatti, F., Pedersen, B. Exercise as an anti-inflammatory therapy for rheumatic diseases-myokine regulation. (2015). *National Review of Rheumatology, 11*, 86-97. https://doi.org/10.1038/nrrheum.2014.193

Blundell, J. E., Gibbons, C., Caudwell, P., Finlayson, G., & Hopkins, M. (2015). appetite control and energy balance: impact of exercise. *Obesity Reviews, 16*, 67-76. https://doi.org/10.1111/obr.12257

Bonini, L., Rotunno, C., Arcuri, E., & Gallese, V. (2022). Mirror neurons 30 years later: implications and applications. *Trends in cognitive sciences, 26*(9), 767-781. https://doi.org/10.1016/j.tics.2022.06.003

Buffey, A.J., Herring, M.P., Langley, C.K. *et al.* The Acute Effects of Interrupting Prolonged Sitting Time in Adults with Standing and Light-Intensity Walking on Biomarkers of Cardiometabolic Health in Adults: a Systematic Review and Meta-analysis. *Sports Med* 52, 1765-1787 (2022). https://doi-org.uos.idm.oclc.org/10.1007/s40279-022-01649-4

Campbell, K. L., Zadravec, K., Bland, K. A., Chesley, E., Wolf, F., & Janelsins, M. C. (2020). The Effect of Exercise on Cancer-Related Cognitive Impairment and Applications for Physical Therapy: Systematic Review of Randomized Controlled Trials. *Physical Therapy, 100*(3), 523-542. https://doi.org/10.1093/ptj/pzz090

Carter, L. G., Lewis, K. N., Wilkerson, D. C., Tobia, C. M., Ngo Tenlep, S. Y., Shridas, P., ... & Pearson, K. J. (2012). perinatal exercise improves glucose homeostasis in adult offspring. *American Journal of Physiology-Endocrinology and Metabolism, 303*(8), E1061-E1068. https://doi.org/10.1152/ajpendo.00213.2012

Chennaoui, M., Arnal, P. J., Sauvet, F., & Léger, D. (2015). sleep and exercise: a reciprocal issue. *Sleep Medicine Reviews, 20,* 59-72. https://doi-org.uos.idm.oclc.org/10.1016/j.smrv.2014.06.008

Cheval, B., Radel, R., Neva, J. L., Boyd, L. A., Swinnen, S. P., Sander, D., & Boisgontier, M. P. (2018). Behavioral and neural evidence of the rewarding value of exercise behaviors: a systematic review. *Sports Medicine, 48,* 1389-1404. https://doi-org.uos.idm.oclc.org/10.1007/s40279-018-0898-0

Christensen, R.H., Wedell-Neergaard, AS., Lehrskov, L.L. *et al.* The role of exercise combined with tocilizumab in visceral and epicardial adipose tissue and gastric emptying rate in abdominally obese participants: protocol for a randomised controlled trial. *Trials* **19**, 266 (2018). https://doi.org/10.1186/s13063-018-2637-0

Clauss, M., Gérard, P., Mosca, A., & Leclerc, M. (2021). Interplay between exercise and gut microbiome in the context of human health and performance. *Frontiers in Nutrition,* 305. https://doi.org/10.3389/fnut.2021.637010

Crush, E. A., Frith, E., & Loprinzi, P. D. (2018). Experimental effects of acute exercise duration and exercise recovery on mood state. *Journal of Affective Disorders, 229,* 282-287. https://doiorg.uos.idm.oclc.org/10.1016/j.jad.2017.12.092

Deslandes, A., Moraes, H., Ferreira, C., Veiga, H., Silveira, H., Mouta, R., ... & Laks, J. (2009). Exercise and mental health: many reasons to move. *Neuropsychobiology, 59*(4), 191-198. https://doi.org/10.1159/000223730

Dishman, R. K. (1997). brain monoamines, exercise, and behavioral stress: animal models. *Medicine & Science in Sports & Exercise, 29*(1), 63-74. https://doi.org/10.1097/00005768-199701000-00010

Dunlap, J., & Barry, H. C. (2011). overcoming exercise barriers in older adults. The Physician and Sportsmedicine, 39(1), 69-75. https://doi.org/10.3810/psm.1999.10.15.1073

Ekkekakis, P., Hartman, M. E., & Ladwig, M. A. (2020). affective responses to exercise. *Handbook of Sport Psychology*, 231-253. https://doi.org/10.1002/9781119568124.ch12

Ellingsgaard, H., Hojman, P., & Pedersen, B. K. (2019). exercise and health-emerging roles of IL-6. *Current Opinion in Physiology, 10*, 49-54. https://doi.org/10.1016/j.cophys.2019.03.009

Ganguly, K., & Poo, M. M. (2013). activity-dependent neural plasticity from bench to bedside. *Neuron, 80*(3), 729-741. https://doi.org/10.1016/j.neuron.2013.10.028

Ghafouri-Fard, S., Hussen, B. M., Ganjo, A. R., Jamali, E., & Vataee, R. (2022). A concise review on the interaction between genes expression/polymorphisms and exercise. *Human Gene, 33*, 201050. https://doi-org.uos.idm.oclc.org/10.1016/j.humgen.2022.201050

Gilbert, P. (2015). the evolution and social dynamics of compassion. *Social and Personality Psychology Compass, 9*(6), 239-254. https://doi.org/10.1111/spc3.12176

Gomes-Neto, M., Conceicao, C. S., Carvalho, V. O., & Brites, C. (2013). A systematic review of the effects of different types of therapeutic exercise on physiologic and functional measurements in patients with HIV/AIDS. *Clinics, 68*, 1157-1167. https://doi.org/10.6061/clinics/2013(08)16

Hagger, M. & Chatzisarantis, N. (2008). Self-determination Theory and the psychology of exercise, *International Review of Sport and Exercise Psychology, 1*:1, 79-103, https://doi.org/10.1080/17509840701827437

Hassandra, M., Goudas, M., & Theodorakis, Y. (2015). Exercise and Smoking: A Literature Overview. *Health, 7*(11), 1477-1491. https://doi.org/10.4236/health.2015.711162

Hirvensalo, M., & Lintunen, T. (2011). Life-course perspective for physical activity and sports participation. *European Review of Aging and Physical Activity, 8*(1), 13-22. https://doi.org/10.1007/s11556-010-0076-3

Dinoff, A., Herrmann, N., Swardfager, W., Gallagher, D., & Lanctot, K. L. (2018). The effect of exercise on resting concentrations of peripheral brain-derived neurotrophic factor (BDNF) in major depressive disorder: A meta-analysis. *Journal of Psychiatric Research, 105*, 123-131. https://doi.org/10.1016/j.jpsychires.2018.08.021

Fernández-Lázaro, D., González-Bernal, J. J., Sánchez-Serrano, N., Navascués, L. J., Ascaso-del-Río, A., & Mielgo-Ayuso, J. (2020). physical exercise as a multimodal tool for COVID-19: Could it be used as a preventive strategy. *International Journal of Environmental Research and Public Health, 17*(22), 8496; https://doi.org/10.3390/ijerph17228496

Hansen, E. S. H., Pitzner-Fabricius, A., Toennesen, L. L., Rasmusen, H. K., Hostrup, M., Hellsten, Y., ... & Henriksen, M. (2020). Effect of aerobic exercise training on asthma in adults: a systematic review and meta-analysis. *European Respiratory Journal, 56*(1). https://doi.org/10.1183/13993003.00146-2020

Juan J, Liu G, Willett WC, Hu FB, Rexrode KM, Sun Q. (2017). Whole grain consumption and risk of ischemic stroke: Results From two Prospective Cohort Studies. *Stroke, 48*(12):3203-3209. https://doi.org/10.1161/strokeaha.117.018979

Khorshid Ahmad, T., Acosta, C., Cortes, C., Lakowski, T. M., Gangadaran, S., & Namaka, M. (2016). Transcriptional Regulation of Brain-Derived Neurotrophic Factor (BDNF) by Methyl CpG Binding Protein two (MeCP2): a Novel Mechanism for Re-Myelination and/or Myelin Repair Involved in the Treatment of Multiple Sclerosis (MS). *Molecular Neurobiology, 53*(2), 1092-1107. https://doi.org/10.1007/s12035-014-9074-1

Kouloutbani, K., Venetsanou, F., Markati, A., Karteroliotis, K. E., & Politis, A. (2022). The effectiveness of physical exercise interventions in the management of neuropsychiatric symptoms in dementia patients: a systematic review. *International Psychogeriatrics, 34*(2), 177-190. https://doi.org/10.1017/S1041610221000193

Lally, P., Van Jaarsveld, C. H., Potts, H. W., & Wardle, J. (2010). How are habits formed: modelling habit formation in the real world. *European Journal of Social Psychology, 40*(6), 998-1009. https://doi.org/10.1002/ejsp.674

Lanfranco F, Strasburger CJ (eds): Sports Endocrinology. front Horm Res. Basel, Karger, 2016, vol 47, pp 44-57. https://doi.org/10.1159/000445156

Law, L. L., Rol, R. N., Schultz, S. A., Dougherty, R. J., Edwards, D. F., Koscik, R. L., ... & Okonkwo, O. C. (2018). Moderate intensity physical activity associates with CSF biomarkers in a cohort at risk for Alzheimer's disease. *Alzheimer's & Dementia: Diagnosis, Assessment & Disease Monitoring, 10*, 188-195. (Amst). https://doi.org/10.1016/j.dadm.2018.01.001

Lee, J. H., & Jun, H. S. (2019). role of myokines in regulating skeletal muscle mass and function. *Frontiers in Physiology, 10*, 42. https://doi.org/10.3389/fphys.2019.00042

Lehrskov, L. L., Lyngbaek, M. P., Soederlund, L., Legaard, G. E., Ehses, J. A., Heywood, S. E., ... & Ellingsgaard, H. (2018). interleukin-6 delays gastric emptying in humans with direct effects on glycemic control. *Cell Metabolism, 27*(6), 1201-1211. https://doi.org/10.1016/j.cmet.2018.04.008

Leitzmann, M., Powers, H., Anderson, A. S., Scoccianti, C., Berrino, F., Boutron-Ruault, M. C., ... & Romieu, I. (2015). European code against cancer 4th edition: physical activity and cancer. *Cancer Epidemiology, 39*, S46-S55. https://doi.org/10.1016/j.canep.2015.03.009

Lindig, A. M., McGreevy, P. D., & Crean, A. J. (2020). Musical dogs: a review of the influence of auditory enrichment on canine health and behavior. *Animals, 10*(1), 127. https://doi.org/10.3390/ani10010127

Livingston, G., Sommerlad, A., Orgeta, V., Costafreda, S. G., Huntley, J., Ames, D., Ballard, C., Banerjee, S., Burns, A., Cohen-Mansfield, J., Cooper, C., Fox, N., Gitlin, L. N., Howard, R., Kales, H. C., Larson, E. B., Ritchie, K., Rockwood, K., Sampson, E. L., Samus, Q., ... Mukadam, N. (2017). dementia prevention, intervention, and care. *Lancet (London, England), 390*(10113), 2673-2734. https://doi.org/10.1016/S0140-6736(17)31363-6

Maass A, Duzel S, Brigadski T, Goerke M, Becke A, Sobieray U, et al. Relationships of peripheral IGF-1, VEGF and BDNF levels to exercise-related changes in memory, hippocampal perfusion and volumes in older adults. (2016). *NeuroImage.* https://doi.org/10.1016/j.neuroimage.2015.10.084

Małkiewicz, M. A., Szarmach, A., Sabisz, A., Cubała, W. J., Szurowska, E., & Winklewski, P. J. (2019). Blood-brain barrier permeability and physical exercise. *Journal of Neuroinflammation, 16*(1), 1-16. https://doi.org/10.1186/s12974-019-1403-x

Mohammed, J., Derom, E., Van Oosterwijck, J., Da Silva, H., & Calders, P. (2018). Evidence for aerobic exercise training on the autonomic function in patients with chronic obstructive pulmonary disease (COPD): a systematic review. *Physiotherapy, 104*(1), 36-45. https://doi-org.uos.idm.oclc.org/10.1016/j.physio.2017.07.004

Morres, I. D., Hatzigeorgiadis, A., Stathi, A., Comoutos, N., Arpin-Cribbie, C., Krommidas, C., & Theodorakis, Y. (2019). Aerobic exercise for adult patients with major depressive disorder in mental health services: a systematic review and meta-analysis. *Depression and Anxiety, 36*(1), 39-53. https://doi.org/10.1002/da.22842

Moore SC, Lee IM, Weiderpass E, Campbell PT, Sampson JN, Kitahara CM et al. (2016) Association of leisure-time physical activity with risk of 26 types of cancer in 1.44 million adults JAMA Intern, 176:816-825. https://doi.org/10.1001/jamainternmed.2016.1548

Moustafa, A. A., Crouse, J. J., Herzallah, M. M., Salama, M., Mohamed, W., Misiak, B., ... & Mattock, K. (2020). depression following major life transitions in women: a review and theory. psychological reports, 123(5), 1501-1517. https://doi.org/10.1177/0033294119872209

Osilla EV, Safadi AO, Sharma S. Calories. [Updated 2022 Sep 12] In: StatPearls [Internet]. Treasure Island (FL): StatPearls Publishing; 2022 Jan-. Available from: https://www.ncbi.nlm.nih.gov/books/NBK499909/

Park, J. H., Moon, J. H., Kim, H. J., Kong, M. H., & Oh, Y. H. (2020). sedentary lifestyle: overview of updated evidence of potential health risks. Korean Journal of Family Medicine, 41(6), 365-373. https://doi.org/10.4082/kjfm.20.0165

Pouwels, S., Stokmans, R. A., Willigendael, E. M., Nienhuijs, S. W., Rosman, C., van Ramshorst, B., & Teijink, J. A. (2014). Preoperative exercise therapy for elective major abdominal surgery: a systematic review. International Journal of Surgery, 12(2), 134-140. https://doi.org/10.1016/j.ijsu.2013.11.018

Petersen, A. M. W., & Pedersen, B. K. (2005). the anti-inflammatory effect of exercise. Journal of Applied Physiology, 98(4), 1154-1162. https://doi.org/10.1152/japplphysiol.00164.2004

Reimers, A. K., Wagner, M., Alvanides, S., Steinmayr, A., Reiner, M., Schmidt, S., & Woll, A. (2014). proximity to sports facilities and sports participation for adolescents in Germany. PloS One, 9(3), e93059. https://doi.org/10.1371/journal.pone.0093059

Ruple, A., MacLean, E., Snyder-Mackler, N., Creevy, K. E., & Promislow, D. (2022). dog models of aging. *Annual Review of Animal Biosciences, 10*, 419-439. https://doi.org/10.1146/annurev-animal-051021-080937

Saunders, T. J., McIsaac, T., Douillette, K., Gaulton, N., Hunter, S., Rhodes, R. E., ... & Healy, G. N. (2020). sedentary behavior and health in adults: an overview of systematic reviews. *Applied Physiology, Nutrition, and Metabolism, 45*(10),

S197-S217. https://doi.org/10.1139/apnm-2020-0272

Spalding, K. L., Bhardwaj, R. D., Buchholz, B. A., Druid, H., & Frisén, J. (2005). retrospective birth dating of cells in humans. *Cell, 122*(1), 133-143. doi: 10.1016/j.cell.2005.04.028.

Stanford, K. I., Lee, M. Y., Getchell, K. M., So, K., Hirshman, M. F., & Goodyear, L. J. (2015). Exercise before and during pregnancy prevents the deleterious effects of maternal high-fat feeding on metabolic health of male offspring. *Diabetes, 64*(2), 427-433. https://doi.org/10.2337/db13-1848

Time to get off the couch, WHO warns, as 500 million risk developing chronic disease, (2022). Retrieved on 15 December, 2022, from: https://news.un.org/en/story/2022/10/1129662

Terry, P. C., Karageorghis, C. I., Curran, M. L., Martin, O. V., & Parsons-Smith, R. L. (2020). Effects of music in exercise and sport: A meta-analytic review. *Psychological Bulletin, 146*(2), 91–117. https://doi.org/10.1037/bul0000216

Thune, I., Brenn, T., Lund, E., & Gaard, M. (1997). physical activity and the risk of breast cancer. *New England Journal of Medicine, 336*(18), 1269-1275. https://doi.org/10.1056/nejm199705013361801

Rahman, M. S., Helgadóttir, B., Hallgren, M., Forsell, Y., Stubbs, B., Vancampfort, D., & Ekblom, Ö. (2018). cardiorespiratory fitness and response to exercise treatment in depression. *BJPsych Open, 4*(5), 346-351. https://doi.org/10.1192/bjo.2018.45

Reimers CD, Knapp G, Reimers AK. (2009). Exercise as stroke prophylaxis. dtsch Arztebl Int., 106(44):715–721. https://doi.org/10.3238/arztbl.2009.0715

Safdar, A., Bourgeois, J. M., Ogborn, D. I., Little, J. P., Hettinga, B. P., Akhtar, M., ... & Tarnopolsky, M. A. (2011). endurance exercise rescues progeroid aging and induces systemic mitochondrial rejuvenation in mtDNA mutator mice. *Proceedings of the National Academy of Sciences, 108*(10), 4135-4140. http://www.pnas.org/cgi/doi/10.1073/pnas.1019581108

Taliaz D, Stall N, Dar DE, Zangen A. (2009). Knockdown of brain-derived neurotrophic factor in specific brain sites precipitates behaviors associated with depression and reduces neurogenesis. Mol Psychiatry. 15(1):80-92 https://doi.org/10.1038/mp.2009.67

Teixeira, André L.; Fernandes, Igor A.; Vianna, Lauro C. (2020). Cardiovascular Control During Exercise: The Connectivity of Skeletal Muscle Afferents to the Brain. *Exercise and Sport Sciences Reviews, 48*, Issue 2, p. 83-91. https://doi.org/10.1249/jes.0000000000000218

Thangudu, Suresh, Fong-Yu Cheng, and Chia-Hao Su. 2020. "Advancements in the Blood-Brain Barrier Penetrating Nanoplatforms for Brain Related Disease Diagnostics and Therapeutic Applications", *Polymers, 12*, no. 12: 3055. https://doi.org/10.3390/polym12123055

Tiozzo E, Youbi M, Dave K, Perez-Pinzon M, Rundek T, Sacco RL, et al. (2015). Aerobic, resistance, and cognitive exercise training poststroke. *Stroke. 46*:2012-6 https://doi.org/10.1161/strokeaha.114.006649

Woerle, H. J., Albrecht, M., Linke, R., Zschau, S., Neumann, C., Nicolaus, M., ... & Schirra, J. (2008). Importance of changes in gastric emptying for postprandial plasma glucose fluxes in healthy humans. *American Journal of Physiology-Endocrinology and Metabolism, 294*(1), E103-E109. https://doi.org/10.1152/ajpendo.00514.2007

WHO (2020). WHO guidelines on physical activity and sedentary behavior. Retrieved on 11 November, 2022 from: https://www.who.int/publications/i/item/9789240015128

Wohlrab, M., Klenk, J., Delgado-Ortiz, L., Chambers, M., Rochester, L., Zuchowski, M., ... & Jaeger, S. U. (2022). The value of walking: a systematic review on mobility and healthcare costs. *European Review of Aging and Physical Activity*, *19*(1), 31. https://doi-org.uos.idm.oclc.org/10.1186/s11556-022-00310-3

Xing, Y., Yang, S. D., Dong, F., Wang, M. M., Feng, Y. S., & Zhang, F. (2018). The beneficial role of early exercise training following stroke and possible mechanisms. *Life sciences*, *198*, 32-37. https://doi.org/10.1016/j.lfs.2018.02.018

Yamanaka, Y., Honma, K. I., Hashimoto, S., Takasu, N., Miyazaki, T., & Honma, S. (2006). Effects of physical exercise on human circadian rhythms. *Sleep and Biological Rhythms*, *4*(3), 199-206. https://doi-org.uos.idm.oclc.org/10.1111/j.1479-8425.2006.00234.x

Yue, Y., & Quinlan, P. T. (2015). Appraising the role of visual threat in speeded detection and classification tasks. *Frontiers in Psychology*, *6*, 755. https://doi.org/10.3389/fpsyg.2015.00755

Zhao, H. X., Zhang, Z., Zhou, H. L., Hu, F., & Yu, Y. (2020). Exercise training suppresses Mst1 activation and attenuates myocardial dysfunction in mice with type one diabetes. *Canadian Journal of Physiology and Pharmacology*, *98*(11), 777-784. https://doi.org/10.1139/cjpp-2020-0205

About the Author — Acknowledgements

Quality of life, together with the factors that enhance it, has been at the heart of Dr Manos Georgiadis's personal journey since he first became aware of himself. He has been in this field for thirty years, advocating important factors in improving quality of life.

In his teenage years he was a swimmer of Ilysiakos (Athens, Greece), winning national victories, breaking national records, and participating in competitions as a member of the national team in international and European swimming events. He started his undergraduate studies at the Department of Physical Education and Sports Sciences (TEFAA) of the National and Kapodistrian University of Athens. After working as a collaborator of the Laboratory of Sport Psychology and Kinetic Behavior at the Kapodistrian and National University of Physical Education and Sport, he continued his postgraduate studies at the University of Exeter, UK, in the field of Exercise and Sport Psychology; the first postgraduate program in the UK and Europe to focus on this subject. He followed that with a PhD at Loughborough University (UK), investigating important factors in motivating Greek populations to change exercise and dietary behavior. He completed his studies with the Applied Psychology program at the City University of Seattle, USA, carrying out his internship at the rehabilitation program of KETHEA (Athens; https://www.kethea.gr/en/).

He is also a specialist in Eclectic Psychotherapy (Dr. Phaedra Logotheti), in Post Traumatic Stress Rehabilitation (EMDR), and in the treatment of Eating Disorders (Master Practitioner in Eating Disorders, UK; KEADD, Athens, Greece, https://eating-disorders.org.uk/international/greece/).

He has been a performance, health, and exercise psychologist for more than 30 years, and a Visiting Professor at the Universities of Athens, Thessaly, and Thrace. He currently holds a full-time academic position at the University of Suffolk (UK). As a researcher of performance, exercise, health, and quality of life, he has published many scientific studies and has presented his research papers in European and international scientific conferences. He has been a program leader in the Physical Education course at the Officers' School of the Hellenic Police for seven years, and a Lecturer in European research and training projects.

His life course was influenced by important teachers he had at the primary school (Marasleio Pedagogical Academy; https://bonflaneur.com/en/athens_points/marasleio-college-of-education/), especially Mrs Biniori, Mrs Metallinou, Mr Arvanitakis, Mr Sparos, Mr Koumelas, and Mr Papathanasiou. His inspirations were, and continue to be, the Professors of Sport Psychology and Exercise Psychology, Dr. Ioannis Zervas, Dr. Stuart Biddle, and Dr. Panteleimon Ekkekakis. They are joined by Dr. Spyridoula Vazou-Ekkekakis, Dr. Nektarios Stavrou, and Major General Dr. Panagiotis Lefas.

He would like to thank from the bottom of his heart Mrs. Asimina Kourouni for her company, support, encouragement, and inspiration. For the valuable comments on the text of the book, he expresses his gratitude to Dr. Nikolaos Houtas and Mr. Evangelos Zoubaneas. And of course, to Ms. Sophia Georgiadis for her unique drawings. He also expresses his thanks to Mr Nathan James for his unreserved support in the publication of this book in English.

The path that started with undergraduate studies in sport sciences and physical education evolved into an interest in scientific knowledge around central behaviors linked to everyday quality of life. Gradually, he entered the field of education in physical activity, performance, eating behavior, sleep, breathing, positive emotions, and the autonomic nervous system.

Wherever he may live in the future, he plans to continue writing, educating, and enhancing quality of life in those around him. He authored this book with such responsibility in mind.

www.ingramcontent.com/pod-product-compliance
Lightning Source LLC
Chambersburg PA
CBHW062101270326
41931CB00013B/3172